D1111767

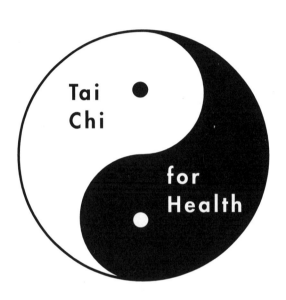

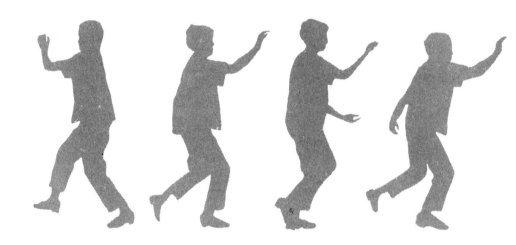

New York   Chicago   San Francisco

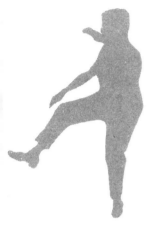

TAI CHI
FOR
HEALTH

Edward Maisel

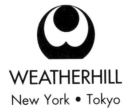

WEATHERHILL
New York • Tokyo

First edition, 1963
First Weatherhill edition, 1998
Second printing, 1999

Copyright © 1963, 1998 by Edward Maisel

Published by Weatherhill, Inc., of New York and Tokyo. Protected by copyright under the terms of the International Copyright Union; all rights reserved. Except for fair use in book reviews, no part of this book may be reproduced for any reason by any means, including any method of photographic reproduction, without permission of Weatherhill, Inc. First published by Prentice Hall, Inc. Printed in the U.S.A.

Library of Congress Cataloging-in-Publication Data:

Maisel, Edward.
    Tai Chi for health / by Edward Maisel
        p.   cm.
    Previously published: New Jersey: Prentice Hall, 1963.
    ISBN 0-8348-0420-4
    1. T'ai chi ch'uan.   I. Title.
RA781.M34   1999
613.7'148—dc21   97-51964
                                                                          CIP

"A fitly born and bred race, growing up in right conditions of outdoor as much as indoor harmony, activity and development, would probably, from and in those conditions, find it enough merely to live—and would, in their relations to the sky, air, water, trees, etc., and to the countless common shows, and in the fact of life itself, discover and achieve happiness—with Being suffused night and day by wholesome ecstasy, surpassing all the pleasures that wealth, amusement, and even gratified intellect, erudition, or the sense of art, can give."

—WALT WHITMAN

To my wife,
Betty Cage

PREFACE TO THE NEW EDITION

As part of their quest to keep in good shape as they enter a new phase of their lives, many baby boomers have taken up regular practice of the enlivening movements described herein. They may be seen everywhere, in groups or as individuals, in parks or in private places, doing their Tai Chi. Newspapers and TV, on their regular beat with news of the boomers, picked up on the story of this widespread phenomenon, and in their reportage specifically mentioned my book as the best basic guide to such activity. Publishers began to inquire. And by curious coincidence the present publisher, quite on its own and unaware of the burgeoning publicity, had already encountered the book and decided the moment was propitious for publishing it once again.

Tai Chi for Health first appeared about a generation ago, and since then, through reprints and new editions, it has established itself as the standard work. In carefully going over the book to prepare for this 1998 version, I was pleased to discover that it can pretty much stand as it was originally written. With the exception of a few minor details and a few additions by way of updating facts, nothing in it has been altered.

A profound debt of gratitude must be expressed here to the many friends and colleagues who have lightened my task in preparing this first American book on classic Tai Chi. In Honolulu it was Thick Poy Young who first awakened me to the exercise. And in San Francisco, Los Angeles, and New York I was in various ways helped by: Shih Lung Liu, Dr. Hui-Ching Lu, Edwin Denby, Wen-shan Huang, Ed Parker, James Wu, Martha Orrick, Da Liu, Kevin Tyler, Yee Chai Cheung, Chung Wo Chee, and Edith Le Clercq. Both Donald Fong and Kenneth Loo were most helpful to me in Honolulu.

To Dr. William C. Hu, Librarian at the Asian Center of the University of Michigan, I should like to acknowledge a special debt for his generously making available the scholarly materials which form the basis of his forthcoming monograph on this history of Tai Chi. From these I have derived the sketch provided in Part Three. Only the brief contemporary account at the conclusion is put together from other sources.

For the clean, serviceable translations of the three classic treatises which are offered in the Appendix, I wish to thank Chao-li Chi, my collaborator upon them.

The San Francisco Tai Chi Chuan Club kindly invited me to a meeting, and we engaged in roundtable consultation long into the night afterwards. The Tai Chi organization in New York's Chinatown, breaking with longstanding precedent, invited me as the first Westerner to their clubroom for a truly unforgettable session of practice.

A number of bibliophiles have kindly placed some rare items at my disposal. Thus it has been possible for me to make a thorough survey of existing Tai Chi manuals in Chinese, old and new.

Also to be acknowledged as contributing helpfully to this 1998 edition of *Tai Chi for Health* are the members of my present class: Alex Schierman, Kiki Smith, Francis Mason, Donna Holly, Senta Driver, Karen von Aroldingen, Christine Redpath.

This book could never have been written without the assistance of my wife, Betty Cage, a Westerner superbly gifted in the practice and richly experienced in the teaching of Tai Chi today. The lesson plan, many subtle pointers in the instructions, and the idea of including transitional movements in the illustrations, all derive from her expert advice.

While later traveling to study with Tai Chi adepts in various countries of the Far East, I noted, with gratification, that some of these novel features are now being incorporated into handbooks published there.

EDWARD MAISEL

March, 1998

CONTENTS

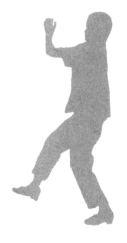

PART I

LEARNING ABOUT TAI CHI

The important health
benefits it offers you

1

Tai Chi:
The what and
the why

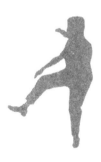

❧   The basic, if slightly embarrass-
ing, truth about exercise is
plain enough: nobody wants to
do the awful stuff. Yet for most of us, calisthenics, that
unwanted addition to the unpleasantries of daily existence,
has remained the only practical way of keeping fit. "Calisthenics," as one report to the nation had the candor to
admit, "most people won't touch with a barbell."

Tai Chi:
A Non-strenuous,
Pleasant Conditioner

Perhaps, then, for many of us the important news
about an ancient Chinese system of exercise which has
excited the interest of medical men and physical educators
is simply this: it affords a deeply pleasurable experience.
Tai Chi Chuan (pronounced *Tie Jee Chwahn* and usually
called Tai Chi for short) has almost nothing in common
with the heavy-breathing, exhausting gyrations of our
own calisthenics. It is an easy-to-do, non-strenuous,
pleasant conditioner.

A growing number of people are adopting Tai Chi as
an essential part of their daily program, like food or sleep
or cleanliness. To them it has become a regular hygienic
practice, no more to be neglected than brushing one's
teeth.

And that, after all, is how exercise must be considered
if it is to prove truly beneficial to your physical and
general well-being. It is not something to be taken up in
spurts, something most often left to the occasional practice
of sport on a weekend, holiday or vacation. Rather, the
consensus of medical authorities emphasizes that if exercise is to do any real and continuing good, it should be

incorporated into everyday life as a natural, unforced activity; it should form a necessary ingredient of your daily routine.

The reason, of course, that this has not generally been the case till now is that what is customarily meant by exercise, or calisthenics, is just too unpleasant, a kind of ordeal in fact, and therefore never to be kept up very long, no matter how firm the initial resolution. In due time, moreover, it also becomes apparent to most people that the supposed benefits to be derived from the usual setting-up exercises, or "daily dozen," are quite unnoticeable or else far too limited for the effort involved.

People who bother at all with the whole business, therefore, take it up with a kind of grim, virtuous determination at first, and then almost without fail drop it in the end. There are always plenty of convincing reasons they can give themselves, such as having no time, or being in such a perpetual rush that they keep forgetting about it. Nothing much happens after that, unless perhaps after a while there is a new resolve and a next time when the same futile process is repeated.

Tai Chi—a Health Secret from Ancient China

But the exercise known as Tai Chi has been done by the Chinese—the inventors and developers of it—faithfully for hundreds and hundreds of years right up to the present day. And among them it has proved not only its durability but also its worth, many times over, through these centuries of widespread practice. It has been put to the practical test of use. Upon the medical history of Europe and America, as we shall later see, it has also had a considerable effect.

"No way of thinking or doing, however ancient," a crusty American individualist, Henry David Thoreau, once wrote, "can be trusted without proof." As Westerners we are bound to hold with Thoreau on this point. Especially perhaps do we have the right to be wary of ancient practices from the East, when we recollect how much nonsense with an Eastern label has got itself accepted by the credulous among us in the name of highbrow esotericism.

Tai Chi's Benefits Endorsed by Medical Authorities

What is perhaps most to be remarked, therefore, by modern Western students of Tai Chi is the way in which it would seem to accord with both biomechanical and neurophysiological concepts and principles in the light of present knowledge. It jibes with the nature of sensorimotor behavior as we understand it today. Such proof is bound to impress us as much as the evidence of continued use dating from antiquity.

Not surprisingly, then, one specialist in internal medicine, Dr. Charles W. Bien, in formulating his opinion of Tai Chi, has stated, "As a doctor, I consider such exercise as one of the best methods of preventing illness and of promoting good health." Dr. Bien, who is on the staff of the Kaiser Foundation Hospital at Vallejo, California, perhaps took note of the regularity with which this exercise—because it is so pleasurable—is practiced, when he commended it to all "for better health, greater happiness and more successful living."

This book takes off from no mumbo-jumbo or cultist platform, but from the pragmatic viewpoint of what is now understood in such fields as anatomy, physiology and psychology. Unless one is interested in doing so, one need not adopt any esoteric doctrines or occult beliefs in order to profit immensely from this tried and true, centuries-old manner of exercise. Anyone who should happen to be thus interested, however, or who merely wishes to take a look at the philosophical background of the long-before, original Taoism—which had later an indirect influence upon the development of Tai Chi—may fortunately find just what he is looking for in a first-rate popular book, *The Parting of the Way* by Holmes Welch, who expounds this matter in intelligent up-to-date terms.

In point of historic fact, for the greatest number of Chinese themselves, who have practiced it for so many hundreds of years and who still—both in Taiwan and in mainland China—do so today, the exercise is an indispensable adjunct to staying young and in good health, as well as a precious emotional stabilizer. The great majority, that is, have always engaged in it, and do so still, quite without any mystic or religious purpose. It is simply vital hygiene.

About the philosophic tenets of the Taoist movement which gave birth to Tai Chi, therefore, I shall have little enough to say except whatever might practically assist the student in learning the exercise. But it would not be right that my silence in this respect should be construed too complimentarily. For according to Lao-tzu, the nominal founder of Taoism, and referring to the inmost meaning of this philosophy: the man who is silent knows; the man who speaks does not know. The reader impressed by my silence ought at least to consider a third, less flattering possibility unremarked by the great sage-founder: the man who does not speak and who does not know.

The Dangers of Strenuous Physical Activity

Sports and athletics, though a good deal more fun, are, unfortunately for most people, just as unsatisfactory an answer to the question of keeping in good physical condition as the usual forms of calisthenics.

For this there are several reasons. To begin with, except for the professional athlete, our participation in sports and athletic events is too infrequent to sustain us in the continuing fashion required by decent health. Most sports take a sizable amount of time. They cannot very conveniently be pursued through most of the days, weeks, months and years which make up our lives.

The real dangers, moreover, which may be involved in such on-again off-again indulgence in strenuous physical activity are now clearly recognized. When for example a sudden craze for fifty-mile hikes hit the country in 1963, medical authorities at once spoke out against it. "People can endanger themselves," warned the American Medical Association. "We get distressed when people go out and strain themselves."

Such wearing hikes, explained Dr. Leonard I. Gordon, a New York heart specialist, might be excellent if one were used to them as a regular thing. "But to take a man off a sedentary job," Dr. Gordon cautioned, "—to push him out of his swivel chair and on the road—is not." And a former head of the American Heart Association, Dr. J. Scott Butterworth, acknowledged that walking fifty miles might prove no great problem for Boy Scouts, "but it's not very sensible," he urged, "for people who are not used to it."

On the same score Dr. Janet Travell, President Kennedy's physician, had already put in a bad word for the supposed American virtue of "efficiency." It is not only the businessman who sits at a desk the whole week and then plays golf all weekend, according to Dr. Travell, who is asking for trouble. There are also the women who do all their ironing on one day of the week, or who make all their purchases, however heavy the bundles, in a single visit to the supermarket, or who tackle all the household chores, from bathing babies to mopping floors, in one session. There are also the do-it-yourself handymen who spend a sedentary week at the office, and then paint ceilings on Saturdays and Sundays.

To all such paragons of "efficiency," Dr. Travell's message was brief: *Don't!* At best, muscular aches may lie in store for you; at worst, a weakening of the heart.

It is not only for the average passive citizen that the ill effects, or even possible serious harm, of heavy exertion in sports or other types of activity are now accepted. Important voices are also being raised to question the value of strenuous exercise even for those who do happen to be accustomed to it.

The Effect of Exercise on Life Span

Perhaps the most extensive and systematic research project on the whole topic ever to be conducted in this country was on rats, not men, at the University of Miami Medical School under the direction of Dr. Gordon C. Ring, Chairman of the Department of Physiology. Genetic differences among human beings make it almost impossible to evaluate the important question of what effect exercise may have upon the life span. Dr. Ring and his group, therefore, worked with rats inbred for some eighty generations in order to obtain an answer to this question.

It took them several years, while the subjects were being put through their moderate rodent-style calisthenics, but the results did not show anything significant as to whether moderate activity slows the aging processes. What about the other kind, however? What about strenuous exercise in prolonging useful life? "In fact quite the opposite can be shown to be true for heavy work," declares Dr. Ring. "The statistics for boilermakers, blacksmiths and the like," he points out, "clearly show that their life span is less than that of the general population."

Sports Are Not the Answer

The social context in which we are usually obliged to engage in sports adds to the harm they often do us. In his *The Uses of Ineptitude,* Nicholas Samstag suggests that "a large fraction of all men engaging in active sports today would obtain a prompt cease-and-desist order (and many of them would receive it with a secret sigh of relief)" if they were to get a complete physical examination and then give their doctors an honest picture of how they were getting their exercise. With engaging candor Samstag himself offers us a typical picture:

> Two rounds of golf a week (one each on Saturday and Sunday) don't sound like a killing chore until you learn that they are played in an atmosphere of tension in the company of people on whom the player depends for his livelihood, or that they are followed too quickly by too much heavy food and drink or that they're split rounds, rounds in which the foursome stops after the ninth hole for lunch. It is a wry fact that this pernicious habit usually begins because the player feels that 18 successive holes are too many for him—probably a sound observation. But it is a moot question whether the second nine holes of the new regime aren't even worse for him, played, as they usually are, with blood pressure and belly distended by too much alcohol, food and competitive exuberance.

Who is there who could not match the foregoing with a parallel account of the "benefits" too often derived from his own pursuit of fitness through sports, through bowling or riding or billiards perhaps? Who is there who could not do so, that is, if he were able to face the whole subject with such unflinching honesty?

2

How Tai Chi
works wonders
for your health

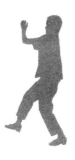

❧ One big shortcoming of most sports is something they have in common with the usual type of calisthenic: too little of the body is exercised. They involve only a limited number of the many possible combinations of muscle groups. Yet good physical development must bring into play the widest variety of such combinations. It is not enough to concentrate upon a few muscle complexes while completely neglecting others which are equally, or even more, important.

Because the movements needed in the majority of athletic activities are seldom comprehensive in this way, they do not provide a symmetrical, all-around conditioning. How often a woman in evening dress is dismayed at the disparity between her well-developed "tennis arm" and her other arm.

Tai Chi: An All-Around Conditioner

It is the unique virtue of Tai Chi as a system of exercise that it makes use of the entire organism. Hands, shoulders, elbows, fists, palms and fingers, abdomen, hips, buttocks, feet, legs, knees, toes, sides of feet and soles—even the eyes—all are brought into play in a series of specific learned patterns of movement called *forms*. And by moving about as these forms prescribe, your breathing is stimulated and assisted as well.

108 Easy Ways to Health —Done Slow and Easy

The forms, 108 in number (many of them repeats or variations, however, of 37 basic actions), are carried out in a definite sequence and can be learned gradually over a planned period of time. Serious students may go on learning to add new and subtle details of movement and coordination.

Tai Chi is characterized by extreme slowness (at first), absolute continuity of movement without break or pause, and a concentrated awareness of what one is doing at all times.

By many persons Tai Chi is never done other than slowly, as slowly as possible. And it does in fact have to be learned that way in the beginning, though later you may do it as rapidly and vigorously as you like. (*See* Tai Chi With Speed, *page 162.*) In this book, which is intended for learning, however, we shall mainly be concerned with the slow practice of it.

Throughout, the body is clothed, loose, and at ease, and all movements contain circles. There is never any straining: Rule Number One is that if it does not feel light and natural, it is wrong. "Comfortable" should be the most frequent and basic word in all learning of Tai Chi. Arms and hands, for example, are gently curved and never held *straight* at the sides, or projected *straight* forward.

Smoothly flowing from start to finish, the exercise is never interrupted, not even for a moment. No poses are struck, no postures held. As each form is approximately completed, the movement already begins to melt and blend into the next form, and so on to the conclusion.

One unchanging tempo is maintained throughout, the slower the better. (Even when you do it speedily you must keep it at the same rate throughout.) The process is compared by one teacher to the slow and even chewing needed for the enjoyment of food. "Without slow chewing," he says, "the flavor of the food is unappreciated . . ." For beginners, it may take 14 minutes to go through the entire calisthenic; after long practice, you can prolong it to nearly twice that.

The obvious analogy here with what we see in slow-motion moving pictures may very well cause us to overlook what is one of the truly notable achievements of Tai Chi as a system of exercise. For most of the action we see in slow-motion movies, it should be remembered, cannot really be performed that slowly. The extreme gradualism of the running which we witness, or of the tennis playing, or diving, or whatever other sport is being exhibited thus, is purely the result of a photographic trick. None of it could in fact be done at such snail's pace. The film has simply been exposed at an accelerated speed, so that when it is projected at a normal rate the movement on it seems to proceed with all the zip of molasses.

Tai Chi as we shall see further in the next chapter is a masterpiece of body engineering. With its cool and knowledgeable command of how balance and locomotion are continually being interwoven, it effects a most original and astonishing interplay of these two elements. One result, and a distinguishing mark of the ancient system, is that as you acquire the necessary skill to do so, the movements in it—unlike those manufactured in the slow-motion films—can actually be carried out with infinite slowness.

Not a Dance or a Performance

Though fascinating to watch, Tai Chi is not a dance or any kind of performing art. It is neither accompanied by music nor executed in accordance with any musical rhythm. The important thing is to perform the exercise as a regular habit, at least once a day and preferably twice— perhaps on rising in the morning and before going to bed at night. Nothing whatever in the way of athletic equipment or apparatus is needed. It can be done quietly in an unseen corner any time relaxation is wanted.

No Special Clothing or Equipment Needed

Note: street clothes, office clothes, any clothes, are fine. No special apparel is required. Always before you start Tai Chi, however, be sure to loosen and unfasten your garments so as to feel quite comfortable. Unbutton your shirt collar, open your belt, unzip the side of your blouse, and so on. As much as you can, allow yourself thus to be more free in moving about and less confined and hampered in your breathing.

In a land of complicated gymnastic machines and of whole wardrobes of special costume for physical training, we do not have to feel ourselves alien in this unelaborate Tai Chi approach to calisthenics. There is sound American precedent for it. The author of *Little Women*, Louisa M. Alcott, long championed a simple unloosening of clothes as the important preliminary to healthful exercise. In one novel of hers, published in 1874, her hero Dr. Alex, instituting a program of exercise for his niece Rose, enjoins her to make the necessary clothing adjustments if she would profit from the curriculum he has devised for her.

"That belt is too tight!" Dr. Alex urged Rose, "unfasten it, then you can take a long breath without panting so."

There is only one exception to the rule that anything may be worn during Tai Chi. It is physically *not* possible to do the exercise in high heels. Women may change into any kind of slippers or low-heel shoes when practicing. Men's shoes are always suitable.

Practice Anywhere

Tai Chi can be carried out in almost any size apartment or office. (When the weather permits, doing it outdoors will provide the additional benefit of fresh air.) An expert can go through the whole thing in an area four feet by four feet.

While serving as staff physician at Sing Sing prison, Dr. Alexander Shaanan became an ardent student of Tai Chi. For his patients, the convicts at Ossining, the circumscription of space was an important factor in their physical rehabilitation.

The Breath of Life

Breathing as an exercise will be far from neglected in your practice of Tai Chi. Indeed it will be involved in all 108 forms from first to last. Rather than being conducted as an isolated activity in the form of special breathing exercises, however, it is coordinated with the movement throughout. Therefore you will not have to pay any particular attention to it for a long time.

The real importance of sound respiration, or good breathing, is fully recognized in current medical practice. Unfortunately this practical acceptance is obscured or mixed up in the popular mind with all manner of superstitions, myths and magical claims. It would be hard to find any topic connected with health that is encrusted with so much fakery and cultism.

There is, for example, the Breatharian movement which has its headquarters in Maitland, Florida. Eating, say the Breatharians, is the cause of death. Almost every kind of food whether meat, vegetables, cereals, or legumes, is poison. Fruits and berries are fairly harmless but even living on these is merely a step towards the true goal, which is a diet of air alone. When you can do that and get your full nourishment from breathing without having to eat anything at all any more, you will be able to live for hundreds of years. In fact if you really make a go of this complete air menu, promise the Breatharians, you will become immortal.

The Benefits of
Good Breathing

The true benefits of good breathing are quite extraordinary enough and do not require all this highflown silliness. For as the *Encyclopedia Britannica* remarks, respiration is a process involved with nothing less than "the chemical basis of life." And your cells, like those of all animals, obtain most of their energy from the burning of foods in this process.

It is the function of breathing to burn up the waste material constantly being formed by the body. As a result of good respiration, your blood will go coursing through your body in a more purified stream. There will be an important effect upon the movement of the lymphatic fluids. Your muscles everywhere will be better nourished, and your vital organs as well. There will be improvement in your digestion and metabolism. The waste materials of your body will be more effectively carried off. Your circulation will show the boost it has received.

All your vocalization is affected. When you talk, sing, or laugh, you are not only using your lips, tongue, jaws and mouth, but your breathing machinery as well. In recent times, some of those who have suffered a total loss of voice through physical mishap have even learned to speak again, completely through management of their breath.

Also, more and more is being said today about the intimate relationship between breathing and the state of your mind and emotions. "My breath stopped!" is a familiar expression to all of us, showing the connection in a case of excitement or fear. John Perceval, son of a Prime Minister of England, during the nineteenth century wrote an account of three years of severe mental derangement from which he had finally emerged. In his book, Perceval commented on how good breathing served to "change the whole complexion of my thought and the tenor of my desires."

A saintly Catholic priest of the eighteenth century, Father Joseph Surin, had presented a more dramatic experience. After bringing tranquility to a convent of badly disturbed nuns, Father Surin himself as a result of his arduous labors fell into a state of melancholy which lasted for several years. When he finally came out of this dark period of gloom and despair, the first sign of his return to normal life was a change for the better in his breathing.

The Frog Pond, an autobiography by a woman of our own time, tells how after years of great emotional suffering her ultimate recovery coincided with a new improvement in her breathing.

In an interview on the things needed for happiness, Dr. Paul Goodman, an analyst and widely read social critic of the present day, placed good breathing at the top of the list. For real happiness, declared Dr. Goodman, you need this even more than money, sex or friends.

How Tai Chi Helps You Breathe

Taking a deep breath, as so many believe, does not constitute a breathing exercise. Actually, the way you exhale is of equal importance to the way in which you inhale. When you exhale properly you are doing something every bit as important for your body's health as when you take in oxygen by inhaling.

Each time you begin Tai Chi, as you stand there quietly, try for a good exhalation before starting. Breathe out deeply, without straining. This will both stimulate and relax you. Then initiate your first movement on the inhalation which naturally follows. Before beginning any physical work, for example before picking up a physical object, do the same thing. You will find that it makes the task easier.

At first and for a long time do not give any thought to the question of which movements to inhale on and which to exhale on. In some cases, even at the start, the movements themselves will pretty much decide that for you. It would, for example, be hard to do anything but inhale on the very wide opening-out movement in the first Plate, page 85. Nor could we easily do anything but exhale on the closing-in movement which then directly follows it, Plate 2, page 85. Some advanced students may later wish to work out a specific breathing pattern of their own to be followed consistently throughout the whole of Tai Chi every time they do it. Others prefer to continue with their immediate response to the breathing requirements entailed by each form as they move through it.

Both your breathing in and your breathing out during this exercise should take place through the nose. *Shut Your Mouth, and Save Your Life* was the title of a book published in 1875 by an English traveler to North and South America who had been much impressed by the way Indian mothers always closed their babies' mouths, even when the infants slept, so as to encourage the habit of breathing through the nose. Your mouth, at least during the times you practice Tai Chi, should also be gently closed—but *not clamped*. The facial muscles around your mouth ought to be just as relaxed as the rest of you.

Do not deliberately "sniff" or "suck in" the air. There is no necessity for that. Simply allow your breathing to take place in accord with your expanding, decreasing, ever-changing needs as you move about in so many different ways. If you are one of those people who just at the thought that you are doing exercise feels obliged to "sniff" or "suck in" the air purposely as you go along, it might be a good idea to remind yourself now and again of one solid fact: atmospheric pressure. Wherever inside you there is an opening to be reached, the pressure of the air upon you due to the weight of the earth's atmosphere—which runs about 14.69 pounds per square inch—is more than sufficient to do the trick. You can be filled with air by this pressure in exactly the same way that it fills a pair of bellows when the handles are drawn apart. You do not have to work at pulling in the air.

This is not, of course, to say that deep breathing will not occur, but the manner in which it does is one of Tai Chi's chief glories. If you suddenly begin breathing deeply —that is, not just with the lungs, but also with the diaphragm, your inmost breathing center—you may find that your system is not accustomed to it. You might soon experience what has been described as an "oxygen jag," which is less expensive than brandy but has pretty much the same effect.

Explaining that such heady upsets "may easily lead to mental disturbances of the most dangerous kind," an eminent Western devotee of Yoga, Christopher Isherwood, states that under no circumstances should the Hindu method be undertaken without "the constant supervision of an experienced teacher." For those who encourage others to attempt it, whether through books or popular lessons, without such expert and continual direct supervision, Mr. Isherwood has very harsh words indeed. They can only be "described as criminals," he declares.

Avoid the "Oxygen Jag"

Instead of resorting, then, to any special exercises which result in "jags," you are going to adjust to deeper breathing through the gradual coordination of your breathing movements with your body movements. That is what takes place with continued practice of Tai Chi. By this process you gently stimulate and encourage the use of the diaphragm.

In time as you go along, you might find yourself emitting deep sighs and yawns. Do not suppress them, or any other heavy breathing sounds you might find yourself making: they come involuntarily and are excellent signs that you are responding properly to the 108 forms.

Exercise, done in a properly relaxed way, is the best possible stimulator and regulator of breathing. On this account, Tai Chi receives high commendation from a veteran clinical authority on breathing. Elizabeth Beit did most of her work as respiratory technician in the field of physical medicine, serving through nearly a decade at such places as the Neurological Institute of New York (a unit of the Columbia-Presbyterian Hospital) and the New York State Rehabilitation Hospital at West Haverstraw. She assisted on cases of polio, arthritis, neurological deficiency and other medical problems. Miss Beit declares:

> The majority of people today are shallow chest-breathers. And to offer them the techniques of Yoga or any other kind of respiratory sophistication does not make much sense. They are all in the kindergarten of breathing. What most of them need before anything else is to become aware of their diaphragm and gradually to develop it in the respiratory function.
> What I should call the orchestration of breathing with movement in Tai Chi is magnificent for this purpose. The way in which breathing supports movement, while movement reinforces breath-

ing, is also something that may continuously be discovered by the man or woman who keeps on with the Chinese exercise.

Breathing is not something to be superimposed upon experience. It should arise, as in Tai Chi, in answer to the infinitely precise exigencies of experience.

3

Other health benefits of Tai Chi

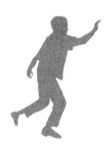

❧ *How to Live 100 Years* is the title which has been given to a collection of three treatises by Luigi Cornaro, a sixteenth-century Italian nobleman. In his merry pages Cornaro celebrates the undiminished good health which he still enjoyed at the age of 99, and makes mention of his continued physical activity.

Outside of a few hints like Cornaro's, the importance of exercise for those past early youth has been neglected in Western culture.

In 1963, the American Medical Association, having appointed a special Committee on Aging to take a good hard look at the nation's senior citizens, announced it was high time to take a fresh approach to the question. One very strong conclusion deduced from the Committee's three-year survey was that old people greatly need activity.

Age Is No Barrier

The uses, past and present, that have been made of the system known as Tai Chi provide an illuminating story. Old persons are as capable of this slow-moving exercise as the young; the refreshment produced by the soothing movements is, if anything, more exhilarating to them. A modern handbook issued on Taiwan, written by an 86-year-old teacher, is illustrated by photographs of the author demonstrating the full spectrum of all the forms with easy perfection.

Visitors returning from Hong Kong or Singapore talk of the elderly men and women seen performing their Tai Chi exercises daily in the parks. The photographs of Henri Cartier-Bresson, as well as a vivid documentary, *Behind the Great Wall*, filmed in Communist China, show that people there still engage in the traditional Tai Chi pursuit of fitness. And this pursuit was highlighted during the historic U.S. mission, in 1972, when millions of Americans watched it on TV direct from China.

In Edgar Snow's survey of earlier Communist China *The Other Side of the River,* describing a visit to Shanghai, he recounts:

> At seven o'clock I went down to walk in the Bund gardens which were already well populated. Eager young and middle-aged people were doing their tai chi chuan steps. . . .

In Peking, Snow found hotel servants doing Tai Chi during their idle moments. The aged headwaiter at the Hsin Chiao, the hotel where he was staying, could be seen out on the terrace going through the exercise every morning at six-thirty. "It's good," the old man told him one morning at breakfast, "for personal contradictions."

A Way to Remain Youthful

Tai Chi was, in fact, originated and developed in an almost gerontological spirit among the early Taoists, a movement not only involved with a desire to realize the magnificent potential of the human body, but also with an obsessive quest to prolong youthfulness. Muscles which are not used, the Taoists understood, tend to atrophy—and this withering of inactive muscles constitutes a significant part of the aging process. As stagnant water results in contamination, they felt, so too must the unexercised body cause all manner of physical distemper: the thing to do, therefore, was to move it about in such a way as to stimulate the blood and to encourage breathing.

Evolved through centuries of practical experimentation with anatomy, physiology, and mechanics, the Taoist calisthenic ultimately had major impact on Western medicine. "Techniques of medical gymnastics," wrote Joseph Needham, the eminent British biochemist, "generally supposed to have been a gift of eighteenth-century Sweden to Europe, can be shown to arise in fact directly from the practices of early mediaeval Taoists in China." For it has been discovered that the Chinese inspiration reached the Swedish pioneers of Western gymnastic through the elaborate treatise of a French Jesuit missionary. That is why some of the Tai Chi positions seem immediately, though remotely, familiar to doctors seeing them for the first time today.

Now that the original Taoist gymnastic has begun to take popular hold in America, a fresh variety of views is at last being brought to bear on it. For example, many, reared in the biceps-building, dumbbell-lifting creed, believe that fearful prodigies of vigor are required to accomplish any physical good. The Taoists, singularly indifferent to the charm of building biceps, concerned themselves instead with such health factors as body contour, muscle tone, and live skin condition. Can the soft, non-strenuous movements of this Chinese system be regarded as exercise? George Balanchine, great choreographer of our era, at first thought not—till he reached out and tested how the muscles were behaving in a person doing it.

It is precisely this aspect of Tai Chi which now elicits the firm commendation of Professor Dudley Dean Fuller of Columbia University, a biomechanical investigator and a collaborator on the classic text, *Human Locomotion and Body Form.* Just to hold any muscle in tension, explains Dr. Fuller, requires it to produce a force which is of an exercising nature. Thus it is perfectly possible for gentle movements to produce this kind of muscle stimulation and muscle exercise: we do not have to run up and down stairs or lift weights.

An infinitely sophisticated piece of body engineering, Tai Chi makes use of the principle of constantly shifting weight in order to prevent a feeling of strain in any given movement. We may more readily comprehend something of the ingenuity here, suggests Dr. Fuller, if we contrast the two familiar activities of standing and walking on level ground.

Continuous Flowing
Movement Is the Secret

When we are walking at normal speed, the calf muscles are in tension for only a small fraction of the time, and relaxed for most of the rest of the time. On the other hand, if we are standing motionless the calf muscles are in constant tension because our centre of gravity is on a line in advance of the ankle, and the tense calf muscles are what keep us from falling forward. The result is that when we stand without moving we become more tired than when walking along at a leisurely pace. Who has not observed the way a person waiting any length of time at a bus stop almost instinctively begins to walk up and back, instead of just standing there erect and stationary?

Tai Chi proceeds by means of opposing dispositions of body weight patterned in comfortable alternation throughout. That is why, in learning, you will find it easier not to repeat an isolated action over and over again in order to master it. Always include the action as part of the movements that come before and that follow it, thus avoiding any possibility of exhaustion. This continuous sequence of forms you will find less tiring than stopping and repeating any given form, or segment of movement, by itself.

Tai Chi in Three Sections

Tai Chi is divided into three sections. Each stands as a complete unity or small whole by itself in addition to its character as an integral part of the total pattern. One or two of the sections may be carried out alone, then, whenever you find a stray interval in which to do Tai Chi, but have not enough time to follow all the way through. The first section, however, should always be included. (See SHORT TAI CHI, page 161.)

In purpose and design the three sections form a progression. Section One is the simplest. Section Two is somewhat more complicated. And Section Three is the most complex, though by the time it has been reached, with the preceding two in hand, you are quite ready for it. Physically there has taken place a gradual building up, which still mounts through the third section right up to the end.

Then after you have learned all three sections, and can do Tai Chi whole, this same gradual building of your physical self will keep on going indefinitely. That is because with increasing practice you become able to include more and more details in your daily execution of it, you are capable always of incorporating still more of the movement that is contained in the 108 forms.

With your continuing experience of Tai Chi, moreover, comes still another kind of physical improvement. You will find as you go on that you are deriving ever greater exercise from the movements, even apart from new details you may add. Without the slightest overreaching or overextending of any of your body parts—which would nullify one basic principle of the system—all your movements are being done more *fully*.

You may notice for example that your knees are starting to bend more deeply while at the same time the steps you are now taking clearly mesh with the new lowering of your torso brought about by these deeper knee-bends. For the steps are definitely longer than before. Thus the deepening bend of your forward knee still does not—in any violation of Tai Chi rule—extend beyond the toe of your foot. (*See* No. 1 *of the* SIX HELPFUL HINTS, *page 69.*) Muscles are being stretched, becoming more flexible and strengthened as well. In other words, desirable changes are taking place in your body as you go along, improvements in physical functioning that always accompany slow and steady growth in the practice of Tai Chi.

Tai Chi Prevents
Freak Injuries

To Dr. Harvey Kopell, a stimulating new theorist in the field of orthopedics, Tai Chi offers an attractive possibility. It may serve as a daily prophylactic against certain hitherto mysterious types of self-sustained injuries which are becoming worrisomely common.

For example, a woman arising in the morning immediately bends over the sink to wash and as she starts to get up develops an acute pain in the back which renders her unable to straighten herself. Dr. Kopell, who rejects conventionally vigorous exercise as more likely to do harm than good, suggests that the chief feature of all such peculiar sudden injuries is the lack of any gradual preparatory warm-up activity, which he regards as a necessary safety feature for the body.

The chief site of this slow warming-up preparation he locates in the central nervous system, and he declares the warm-up vital not only for improving the level of one's physical performance—as every professional athlete knows —but also for the prevention of these abrupt freak injuries.

Whether or not you may later wish to practice a more rapid Tai Chi, therefore, it should always be carried out as slowly as possible when done in the morning, or after any period of being sedentary.

How to Relax and
Sleep Well

For a different reason the same might apply when you use it in preparing for bedtime. Going to bed in an anxious, worried, nervous, tense or excited frame of mind is the best way to "murder sleep," as Shakespeare said. If you should find yourself in this state, try the calming, settling effect of Tai Chi in its slowest form just before retiring. This will be an effective means of improving your chances for slumber.

Arthritis and Tai Chi

What I have been speaking of, it must be understood, is Tai Chi as a program to help keep your body in the best possible condition. In health you will feel more secure and self-confident than if you are physically fragile. An excellent physical condition is, of course, also among your best safeguards against illness and, should that occur, against complication.

When, however, it comes to the use of Tai Chi or any form of exercise or activity as a therapeutic measure in the treatment of some disease or physical problem, that is very much a matter to be talked over between you and your doctor. Do not prescribe for yourself.

Both exercise and rest form an important part in the treatment of arthritis, for example. But this widely experienced inflammation of the joints has many and varied forms. Only your physician can tell you if exercise is useful in your form of arthritis. Most likely it is.

If You are Overweight

Obesity is another widespread condition, more and more being described today as a disease. Many would agree with Dr. Jean Mayer, Associate Professor of Nutrition at Harvard University's School of Public Health, who is "convinced that inactivity is the most important factor explaining the frequency of 'creeping' overweight in modern Western societies."

Either the individual will have to step up his activity, says Dr. Mayer, or else he will have to go mildly or acutely hungry all his life. However difficult the first course is, surveying the highly mechanized and sedentary conditions of modern life, the Harvard nutritionist reminds us that the second alternative—enduring a lifetime of hunger—is even tougher. Summing up, Dr. Mayer concludes, "Strenuous exercise on an irregular basis, in untrained individuals already obese, is obviously not what is advocated here.

But a reorganization of one's life to include regular exercise adapted to one's physical potentialities is a justified return to the wisdom of the ages."

It is certainly a return to the wisdom of the Chinese ages. Many a Tai Chi instructor has emphasized the value of the classic calisthenic done as a "regular" thing in order to assist with weight distribution.

The famous English novelist Arnold Bennett, writing long before the serious mid-twentieth century concern about weight reduction had set in, told about the brief daily exercises undertaken by an obese friend of his:

> They occupied but seven minutes per day. In three months he had lost thirty pounds avoirdupois. I can vouch for the case. For the man was myself.

If Tai Chi is used to help tackle your weight problem, there may be personal considerations of how much and how vigorously you should practice it. According to the findings of a 1998 research group, the obesity rate has increased by a third since 1980. The group's director says, "Americans are getting so fat that it's incredible."

Other Personal Problems and Diabetes

A third example of the need for specifics in all therapeutic applications of exercise should suffice. Dr. Bernard J. Pisani, Director of the Department of Obstetrics and Gynecology at the St. Vincent's Hospital in New York, has made the striking observation that for many patients who have just undergone surgery, Tai Chi in its primary slow-motion tempo would afford an ideal means for a gradual return to normal activity. But here, as Dr. Pisani cautions, everything must depend upon the nature of the operation performed and upon the patient's general condition.

Dr. Willard Dalrymple, chairman of Princeton University's health department, has pointed out that exercise plays an especially useful role in the regulation of diabetes, or in rehabilitating a man to full activity follow-ing an acute illness. Wherever helpful in such cases, Tai Chi, like any other form of activity, would have to be regulated as to the amount of time spent upon it, and a rough scale established for increasing the length of prac-tice sessions devoted to it.

To correct *specific* physical defects, certain special exercises of a conventional sort are often useful. Apart from these remedial measures of a quite particular nature, it is worth remarking that Tai Chi as general exercise is possible and helpful to many persons who are physically handicapped. Possession of a defect or disability does not necessarily prevent someone from going through the 108 forms. Any of the forms can usually be tailored expertly so as to encompass the specific handicaps of a student, without at the same time upsetting the intricate balance of the calisthenic's structure as a whole.

Benefits the Eyes

Something must be said about the eye movements which constitute a vital part of the 108 forms. For medical thought today is harking back to the early opinion it once strongly held about our not making enough use of our eyes. Consider for example what is called the first full treatment in print of exercise, the *Book of Bodily Exercise* by Cristobal Mendez, a sixteenth-century Spanish physician. Superlative indeed was the distinguished doctor's estimate of the value of exercise in general—"makes everything more perfect"—but what now stands out is the particular emphasis this "most skillful physician" of Seville in 1553 placed upon the eyes, too, as being parts of the body in dire need of exercise.

Surrounded as we are today by vacant stares, by un-seeing orbs on the faces of so many people about us, few can doubt Mendez' essential rightness any more. And how about ourselves (as we "come to" and notice every once in a while)? Do not our own eyes often tend to get "stuck" in our heads instead of roving about freely with whatever activities engage us, playing their full part in our accomplishment of those activities? The viewpoint of an increasing number of eye specialists in fact has been cogently expressed by Dr. Morris Kaplan, a Denver ophthalmologist:

> Eyes, like fingers, hands, arms, feet, legs, brains, and lungs are to be used and the lack of use may do much greater harm than use. People who tell me they are saving their eyes by not using them are doing their eyes a major disservice.

In Tai Chi as a system of making the best use of the whole body this was well understood. Do not, therefore, neglect to carry out the eye movements which are given as part of the regular instructions. Allow your eyes to move as they are directed to in the instructions. See, but *do not stare fixedly:* if the eyes are to follow a hand as it travels upward, just permit them to follow it, as if observing with simple interest or attention.

4

Greater mental powers through Tai Chi

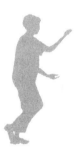

❧ What many medical observers find most striking in Tai Chi is embodied in the opinion of Dr. Walter Thompson, Chairman of Orthopedic Surgery at New York University School of Medicine. He likes Tai Chi as an exercise program "that could be incorporated into one's daily life with real benefit to both the mind and body." The mind? Yes, for the 108 forms cannot be carried out in proper sequence without sensitive concentration upon what one is doing from one moment to the next.

Tai Chi—the Safe Tranquilizer

Your body cannot proceed in automatic dissociation from yourself like a piece of machinery operating on its own while you brood about income taxes, the misfortunes of love, or the menu for dinner. To do this exercise at all, it is absolutely essential to be "with" it; everything else, inevitably, must be excluded. This is the reason why Tai Chi has acquired its curious reputation as the tranquilizer of the East. Among Americans who practice it, it is preferred to any "downer."

When anxious or distracted, persons simply move to a small spot, wherever they may find themselves, and perform their Tai Chi for its calming effect. Erich Fromm in *The Art of Loving* laments that the West has developed so few techniques for this integrative use of the body.

Furnishes Strong Motivation

The lack of a psychological component may indeed finally prove to be the most serious shortcoming in what is customarily meant today by "exercise." For unmotivated physical movements are much more tiring than the same movements performed with interest. Digging and throwing heavy earth for hours on end, a strong man may not feel any particular sense of strain or fatigue. The same man, however, if he is made to go through the identical motions of shovelling, without any shovel in his hands and without heaving any real earth, will give out in a few minutes. It may seem strange at first because, on the face of it, wielding a heavy implement and lifting substantial loads of dirt certainly would appear the more onerous activity.

In the same way, if boys playing "catch" with a baseball are required to go through the motions of throwing and catching a ball, without a ball, they will not keep this up for very long. "This is exactly the factor," S. Arthur Devan wrote, "that makes formal exercise *nervously exhausting*. Many persons who dutifully perform their 'daily dozen' find themselves inexplicably tired all day long afterward."

Never Becomes Dismal or a Dull Habit

The absence of this dismal factor in Tai Chi has won for the exercise an amusing nickname among many of its exponents in America. It came about in the following way.

Sponsored by the New York State Medical Society and the New York City Health Department, during the summer of 1961 I presented the first lecture on Tai Chi to be offered under medical auspices in this country. Shortly thereafter I was invited to give further talks at a number of hospitals and clinics, concerned with its possible applicability in such fields as geriatrics, cardiology, and orthopedics. News of these private lecture-demonstrations came in time to the ears of a journalist, Wadsworth Likely, then an editor of *Newsweek*, who thereupon wrote the first real medical coverage of the ancient calisthenic to appear in any national publication. And it was somewhere during the course of this sizable debut-piece on the subject that Mr. Likely, taking note of the important psychological component in Tai Chi, coined the slogan: "The Thinking Man's Exercise." Directly inspired by his witticism, the *San Francisco Examiner* subsequently ran a whole series of articles under that title, and the nickname seems to have stuck in the newspapers generally, as well as among many students, ever since.

By its very nature, the "thinking man's exercise" can never be a once-and-for-all matter to the people who practice it. Tai Chi cannot settle into a dull habit, something they go through absentmindedly, by rote. It becomes imperative, a kind of necessity, to approach the exercise on every occasion it is done as though going through the 108 forms for the first time. Otherwise you are bound sooner or later to become lost, confused about the subtle details of movement which comprise the forms, or mixed up in trying to follow the proper sequence in which they unfold. This is partly the secret of why the exercise, no matter how often performed, must feel quite spontaneous, as though being always newly explored.

Awakens Your
Mental Powers

This freshness of experience, this feeling of immediacy in whatever we are doing, is a rare thing to most of us. For in our culture, as Dr. Edgar A. Levenson of the William Alanson White Psychoanalytic Institute has shrewdly noted, we have a blind spot. We usually think of time as what is continually passing, as history. The present moment is always a mere transition between yesterday and tomorrow, between the last moment and the next, a kind of bridging from one to the other. How seldom in our culture do any of us "taste" the present moment as just whatever it is (never mind where it came from or where it is headed), only knowing it as completely *now*, as real immediacy. Dr. Levenson recommends:

Recognizing our cultural blind-spots enables us to integrate immediacy into our present psychotherapeutic theories and endeavors, without the uneasiness inherent in feeling we are betraying scientific principle. . . .

For however necessary it may be to keep a grip upon our customary idea of time ever passing, of history always moving, still—according to Dr. Levenson—a direct feel of the present minute, an immediate sense of whatever is happening right now, is "considerably more important to mental health."

One is reminded here of what the old headwaiter at the Peking hotel enigmatically told Edgar Snow about his daily practice of Tai Chi out on the terrace every morning at six-thirty: "It's good for personal contradictions." Neither preoccupation with the past nor worry about the future can find much room in it. Both these twin manifestations of anxiety tend to be eliminated in the full immediacy of having to fulfill, with total awareness and absolutely unbroken continuity of movement, the whole complex of Tai Chi physical-mental requirements: first in this moment, and then in this moment, and then always again in this moment.

Become a "Whole" Person

To trace your gently flowing actions in accordance with the prescribed pattern-series bestows another boon as well. A certain opportunity is thereby offered which can lead to the enrichment of your entire organism. This enricher of the whole person is indeed by some connoisseurs and gourmets of good physical condition esteemed as nothing less than "the crown of the senses," the true distinguishing mark of superb well-being. Whenever we admire the seemingly effortless coordination in the movements of a great athlete or the agile ease and poise of a friend in the way he handles himself in all the ordinary activities of life, we are paying tribute to it.

Clearly evident in people like circus aerialists or

jugglers or sculptors, it is deplorably lacking in a very great number of us. At a UNESCO conference on brain mechanisms and awareness, one speaker even accused the others, in their concern with it, of trying to "unscrew the inscrutable."

It is not really that inscrutable. Most everyone does know something at least about this faculty, the "kinesthetic sense" as it is called. It is often called the "muscle sense" as well, though in fact its sense organs are to be found not only in the muscles but in the tendons and joint membranes also. It is by means of this sense, for example, that even when our eyes are closed we are still aware of the position of every part of our body. It is from this sense that we are always getting knowledge of the gestures we make and of the pressures or tensions anywhere in our body. We use it to assess the range and force of our movements, and also in adapting ourselves to the weight of anything we lift.

Through deliberate practice we can expand the powers we derive from this complicated internal machinery of self-awareness. The virtuoso pianist at the keyboard, the dedicated craftsman working with tools, the expert typist, or the master driver at the steering wheel are ready examples. Each of them, in a given field of activity, has concentrated in his own way upon developing his sensitivity to motion. In ordinary life, such things as our posture and the precision and appropriateness, or the fumbling and clumsiness, of our everyday doings may provide a key to our own kinesthetic refinement—or debauchery.

The "Crown of the Senses"

The "crown of the senses," hardly mentioned at all any more in the fever of recent national fitness rampages, was not always omitted from consideration in the earlier American campaigns for fitness. Taking part in one such effort in 1920, the wise and tireless New England medical educator, Dr. George V. N. Dearborn, crusaded for recognition of the prominent place the kinesthetic sense holds in the life of every individual. "The warp of the sensation-fabric—the personality's dynamic index of its body," was his strong definition of it.

One trouble, as Dr. Dearborn pointed out, is that the too dominant sense experiences of light and color drown out this subtler experience, sometimes so completely that many an adult of intelligence goes through life "wholly ignorant even of the essential existence of these warp-threads in the fabric of our conscious life."

Their importance in a man's living behavior is, unfortunately, not diminished by his ignorance of them. Dr. Dearborn could only feel pity for a man, however excellent his objective mind, who has never developed any phase of motor skill so as to become conscious of this world of submerged sensation. To him such a person must remain always "a clumsy boor, materialistic by nature, loath to become familiar with himself."

"Boors" of this kind the greatest number of us are today. And as an exercise Tai Chi is plainly unique in offering us a large chance to become familiar with ourselves. Steady practice opens up almost limitless avenues toward becoming conscious of the world of submerged sensation within us. The delicate mechanics of the design throughout the 108 forms call for the harmonious interplay of all one's faculties and thereby introduce a novel benefit, the first visible fruit of our growing kinesthetic development: good muscular coordination.

"An excellent self-disciplinary activity for the development of muscular coordination," is how Dr. Allen A. Russek of the Institute of Physical Medicine and Rehabilitation defines his own impression of Tai Chi. As Dr. Russek has pointed out, we have no comparable self-disciplinary system for developing coordination in the West, but must rely chiefly upon various forms of supervised activity.

The Somato-Psychic
Benefits

What it means in actual practice, how it feels, and how it affects one, to carry out as a regular thing this unique, physically-mentally unified calisthenic has not anywhere thus far been more precisely expressed, in my opinion, than by Irmgarde Bartenieff, lecturer in physiotherapy at Columbia University and instructor in that subject at New York University. Her exquisitely perceptive appraisal, because it conveys so much of the true flavor of the experience, is worth giving at some length to illustrate the entire somato-psychic or body-mind nature of the exercise which we have been explaining. In her words:

> Though it is not dance, this solitary ritual of movement transmits the feeling of harmony and rhythm we usually connect with dance movement. It is certainly a far cry from all setting-up exercises Western style. To see these sequences performed, and to do them, provides one with a richly varied kinesthetic experience far beyond feeling one's muscles and joints vigorously stretched. First of all there is the slow sustained rhythm into which the performer has to immerse himself fully in order to maintain it uniformly throughout.
>
> Then the great variety of "shaping" the limbs into constantly varied constellations, making one feel lifted, sinking, expanding and shrinking in succession; and additionally, addressing oneself in various ways to outside space. The whole body is moved through in many ways, but never are extremes of stretching or flexing reached. The whole sequence of 108 variations flows from one movement into the next—with irrefutable logic one is tempted to say—never leaving the orbit of what is comfortable, what "feels well" to move in.
>
> Also never does one move away precariously from the sound balance of all body parts against one another. These facts explain to me the harmonizing and calming effect of Tai Chi, without its ever becoming monotonous. The marvelous balance between continuity of movement and variety of movement-forms requires a full attention and immersion into the whole process. Quite different is all this from the 1-2-3-4 repetitive morning exercises which can so easily be executed in a mechanical manner, and allow the mind to wander.

Advantages Not Found
in Yoga

As research assistant in social psychiatry at Albert Einstein Medical College, Mrs. Bartenieff is conducting pioneering experimental work at Jacobi Hospital in observation and evaluation of movement patterns in the emotionally disturbed. This perhaps lends particular interest to a contrast she draws between Tai Chi and the familiar Hindu techniques which have been popular in this country. She finds:

> It also quite radically differs from Yoga exercises where the emphasis lies in maintaining extremes of body-limb positions in perfectly stable balance, while Tai Chi emphasizes the feel of moving from one state into another. This is therapeutically important when it comes to using body exercise for people with psychological difficulties: the experience of moving may be much more harmonizing than holding extreme positions (yoga), or going through a mechanical routine of exercises.

Some of the Tai Chi instructors in time past remarked upon this basic difference in their own way. They said: Yoga is internal activity and external quiet; Tai Chi is external activity which engenders internal quiet.

There are few of us today, whatever the state of our psychological equilibrium, who could not derive some benefit from this regular experience of complete personal harmony.

5

Tai Chi and your heart

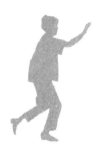

❧ Words of highest praise for Tai Chi are being heard today from medical men struggling at the frontiers of what presently constitutes the Number One health problem in the Western world. Not only to the many who have already developed some form of heart trouble, but also to the great number of people who have begun to concern themselves with the prevention of it, the Chinese calisthenic is, for several reasons, as we shall see, being recommended as a unique measure. Both as a help and as a protection, then, you ought not to overlook its quite special usefulness in this area of prevalent danger.

Heart Trouble
Is Widespread

For most of us by now are aware that, to use the striking language of Dr. Paul Dudley White, elder statesman of cardiology, "the Western world is experiencing the greatest epidemic in all history." In the United States the over-all incidence of coronary disease is 180 per thousand. Apart from those who have been born with some heart defect, it has been reliably estimated that one out of every five North American men before reaching 60 is going to develop coronary trouble. Whether in the form of coronary occlusion or coronary thrombosis, heart attacks are the result of athero-sclerosis, a disease having to do with the condition of the arteries.

Youth is not exempt from its inroads as was frighteningly demonstrated from the autopsies of GI's killed during the Korean Conflict; and the shock of youthful fatality from it is no longer rare. Not only is this disease the first cause of death in America, but it also causes more illness than any other. There are more invalids as a result of it than any other sickness in our time.

Along with investigations of diet, particularly the effect of animal fats and cholesterol, as well as the research devoted to such other possible clues as emotional stress and female hormones, a good deal of attention is now centered upon the importance of regular exercise. This is one factor at least upon which there seems to be almost unanimous agreement.

Lack of Physical Activity
—a Major Factor

In his views, for example, on the prevention of heart disease, Dr. Hans Selye, Director of the Institute of Experimental Medicine and Surgery at the University of Montreal, and famed for his presentation of a comprehensive stress theory, specifically implicates the inactivity which is a part of our life. "The tendency to avoid even the shortest walks by using cars, elevators, etc.," he suggests, may well have been bought at a price. "There is considerable evidence," Dr. Selye continues, "in support of the view that men in physically active jobs have a lower incidence of coronary heart disease in middle age than have men in physically inactive jobs."

Prevention, as well as treatment, is in fact regarded by all medical authority without exception as a major business of the present day. A statement released by the American Heart Association in 1961 took note that the prevention of athero-sclerosis has now become a practical possibility. The manner in which most doctors in the country have reacted to this optimistic possibility was movingly expressed by Dr. George C. Griffith, president of the American College of Cardiology, in a candid declaration of personal policy.

As a practicing physician, could he—Dr. Griffith asked himself—afford to ignore all the data which has been accumulated about heart trouble, awaiting instead some final, certain answer to the problem? Or with full responsibility to his patients, should he not at once institute measures for the prevention and control of it?

Daily Exercise—
a Preventive Measure

"I believe the latter," he affirmed. And among those measures Dr. Griffith stated, "Regular daily exercise with gradually increasing range and scope of effort is clearly reasonable. Exercise prevents sludging and increases fibrinolysins and heparin-like substances." The inclusion of exercise in standard preventive regimen, however, Dr. Griffith took pains to emphasize, meant that physicians truly concerned with heading off coronaries in their patients should prescribe this measure only as a *regular* thing. "The patient," in his words, "should never be allowed to develop into a weekend athlete, crowding all his exercise into an hour or two on Saturday afternoon." It should become, rather, part of his daily "habit pattern."

The strictures upon engaging in volcanic, infrequent bouts of exercise for the purpose of staying in good physical shape, or of maintaining any meaningful kind of fitness, have already been cited.

Particularly strong, however, are the warnings in this regard when a heart condition is involved. It may be recalled that the two specialists who were quoted earlier as representative of the immediate condemnation roused in the medical community by an ephemeral nation-wide fad for fifty-mile hikes happened to be cardiologists. In this branch of medicine, professional sentiment is strong and concerted enough to have made some dent. At least part of the general public has begun to see the light.

Here as a colorful example is the producer of a TV series on *What's Wrong with American Men?* Dramatically, if with considerable exaggeration and the over-simplification customary to the theatre, he gives us his own answer to the question posed by his cycle of programs. "They strive for good health," he says of American men, "so they engage in violent sporadic physical exercise —and wind up with coronaries, shorter lives . . ."

How Tai Chi Benefits
the Heart

The extreme practicality of Tai Chi as a regular day-by-day practice—in contrast to the widespread on-again, off-again indulgence in calisthenics and sports—has now been amply brought out. The discussion, Chapter 3, page 31, shows how ideally in every respect it also fulfills Dr. Griffith's second requirement for exercise beneficial to the heart: how all of its prime characteristics conduce to that "gradually increasing range and scope of effort" which he specifies. The points made there are perhaps worth scanning again in the present context.

Thus a man freshly recuperated from a heart attack, eager but not yet ready to resume his old routine, may early begin his return on that path with Tai Chi, practiced in its slower-than-molasses primary form. Equally, the man who is recovered and back to full normal activity, may practice it with the vigor of lightning-speed, or with whatever may happen to be the maximum rapidity he has been able to attain while keeping an even, unbroken tempo from start to finish.

All such personal questions can be absolutely regulated. How energetic or how melting, and how frequently (how much is too much, or perhaps not enough): in Tai Chi all of that can be—and should be—handily controlled for a heart patient in accordance with his own physician's judgment. Specifics as to amount and extent of activity will naturally differ from one patient to the next, even as they do in some degree among persons with no cardiac complaint.

An important and quite unexpected topic has emerged in recent medical literature dealing with the exercise factor in heart troubles and the prevention of them. Because of its bearing upon Tai Chi as an ideal answer to the total problem, a word or two on this new subject may be in order here.

What Research Revealed

A brilliant piece of research conducted at Western Reserve University, with 39 surgeons themselves as subjects, will most strikingly reveal it to us. Before setting out to perform surgery each of the 39 was ingeniously outfitted with electrodes to give a continuous electrocardiograph of him while he worked, as well as with a cuff to record his blood pressure, and a mask to show how much oxygen he was using. All of them in addition submitted to many kinds of other tests, mental and physical, before they entered the operating room and again after coming out.

From this careful investigation emerged an astonishing result. The surgeons, engaged as they were in such work as cutting and tying small blood vessels, were certainly not doing anything that might be called strenuous labor. *Yet on the average they expended as much energy on their delicate tasks as the average welder or drill-press operator on his heavy job!* At the peak of an operation their heart-beats leapt to an average of 118 a minute. (One surgeon's bounded to 155.) In blood pressure, 23 of them showed no change; 16 had sharp increases.

And the surgeons who put forth the least amount of excess energy, it turned out, were those in the best physical condition. For the most part they were also, according to the psychological tests, those most equable in their ordinary reactions to things.

From the outcome of this research at Western Reserve, Dr. Herman K. Hellerstein, who directed it, drew a firm conclusion. His finding has to do with your circulatory response to any physical activity; in other words, how any kind of exercise or piece of work is going to affect the movement of blood in the vessels of your body, the pumping job that is your heart's chief function.

Your response to such exercise, according to Dr. Hellerstein, depends upon "something" other than the physical effort that is needed to do it. "This 'something' resides in the individual," he states, "and not in the job."

Tai Chi Supplies that
Certain "Something"

By such words we cannot help being reminded of the basic principles of Tai Chi which seemingly take account of the "something" referred to here. We recall, for example, the accent upon *appropriateness* of energy, using no more ever than is required to accomplish any given form (but using that much). Or again we think of the insistence that these 108 forms cannot be accomplished properly, if at all, except in a truly relaxed manner. And of how that manner is encouraged and constantly replenished by the soothing effect of the circular movements, each being always brought to a satisfying rounded completeness before its transition to the next one.

Dr. Allen A. Russek, who has been cited on the topic of muscular coordination, has in effect taken fair account of this "something" component in a remark of his about the Chinese exercise. Tai Chi, he says, has a splendid relaxation potential for "normal people who lead tense, abnormal lives under constant pressure."

On this score Dr. A. T. W. Simeons has questioned even the value of walking as a standard recommendation for persons with heart trouble. He agrees all right that "there can be no doubt that mild, regular exercise is very helpful . . ." But he adds the significant qualification that only "as long as the patient feels he is enjoying himself" is this the case.

"It is useless," advises Dr. Simeons, "to tell a tired, worried businessman to walk twice around the block, just as brooding strolls in the park are not relaxing. There must be enthusiasm and the need to concentrate on something." Tai Chi, as we have seen, demands a certain absorption in order to be done at all.

Tai Chi—the "Wise" Exercise

So is discovered in it another element to endear the Chinese system to those who regard exercise an essential measure with which to meet the new plague we now have to fight, the distinctively modern plague of heart disease which has appeared in our civilization. A cardiologist on the staff of Mt. Sinai Hospital, and author of a treatise presenting a comprehensive technique for analyzing the electromotive forces generated by the heart, Dr. Louis Brinberg formulates his view of the ancient calisthenic:

> Moderate activity is good for most cardiac patients. If it is to be of benefit, however, it should be on a regular basis. Too often patients think that an arduous weekend in the garden or on the golf course, etc., will fill the bill. Exercise taken in this manner is unwise.
>
> One thing I like about Tai Chi is that it is meant to be performed on a regular basis. Another thing that impresses me is that it stresses the gradual approach. Little by little the patient is given a chance to achieve as much as he can within the limits set by the course of his illness. He can eliminate the risk of over-doing en route to these limits and get there without undue effort.
>
> It will be interesting to see what can be done with this exercise when it is used as an adjunct to the usual therapy of cardiac patients.

6

Relaxation and relief from body aches and pains

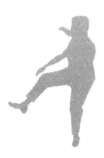

❦ "Posture follows movement like a shadow," wrote Sir Charles Sherrington, the great experimental neurophysiologist. Indeed the relationship between the two works both ways. Our usual habit of carrying ourselves has a great influence upon the way we perform every one of our activities.

The reverse, however, is also true. Our bodily alignment is influenced by the kind of movements we continually make. The man who works bent over something in a large industrial plant or at an agricultural job, as well as the business man slumped in an office seat, is going to exhibit the results of his customary daily movements upon his body.

How are we to get out of this vicious circle if we wish to do something about our posture? For the way we hold ourselves as we move will tend to diminish the effects of those very exercises which we practice in order to improve our bearing. At the same time it is often the case that the movements themselves may be quite without any helpful effect in building posture.

The early inventors of Tai Chi came to grips with the dilemma in a decisive manner. They specified a definite position to be maintained throughout the entire exercise. On the one hand it was intended to facilitate the movements; and on the other, the movements all being complementary to it, were intended to reinforce the position. In this way, through the mutual interreaction of posture and movement, the likelihood of some effectual carry-over into one's daily comportment seemed best insured. And, as we shall see in a moment, certain important benefits both to our general appearance and to our health would follow.

How to Relax the
Entire Body

Relaxation of the entire body, as we already know, is the first part of this specified posture for doing Tai Chi. Here is the second part: most of the time that you are doing the exercise, your head, neck and torso will be in a vertical line, and that line will be straight up-and-down to the floor. This is your "Tai Chi trunk," as it is sometimes called.

Keeping head, neck and torso in a line always perpendicular to the floor does not in the least cancel the first requirement of being totally relaxed. "Posture" here does not imply the same thing as the sergeant's gruff bark of "Ten-shun!"

So dismiss from your mind any images of the marching gray line at West Point or the prancing chorus line at Radio City Music Hall. Beyond the parade ground and the proscenium, for that matter, even the cadets and the Rockettes do not hold onto these strenuously maintained body attitudes. In the ordinary work of sitting, walking and living they drop the elevated chest and the forward curvature of the spine with its accompanying hollow in the back. The effort to hang onto military posture is conscious and continuous, and involves both mental and physical fatigue. Since your freedom of chest movement is held in check it also interferes with breathing, which contributes further to your tiredness.

Become a Marionette

The position kept through most of Tai Chi is simply a vertical alignment, comfortably relaxed, of head, neck and torso. Chinese teachers of the past have used two pictures to illustrate it. In the first of these, they speak of your body as a tree: the trunk is straight and strong, but the roots (the legs) and the branches (the arms) curve and undulate and do various things, always supported by the straight strong trunk.

Be careful, however, not to think of the tree as being stiff or rigid. Your neck for example, though in a line with your head and torso, must always be freely movable, ready to turn in any direction, left, right, or way around. It cannot swivel easily as required to by the instructions if there is any tautness in it. Waist movements are also of the utmost importance, and there should be no rigidity to prevent you from turning at the waist.

The second picture which Tai Chi teachers have offered is a good one to keep in mind. Become a marionette, they suggest. Feel that you are dangling, suspended from a control-wire attached at the top-center of your head. With this concentrated balance of your weight distribution, you will also feel like a marionette in the lightness and ease with which you are able to move about.

Whenever you notice that you are tilted forward or backward to any degree, thus losing the always-vertical of your "Tai Chi trunk," there is a simple remedy for it. Sometimes increasing your step is what will bring you upright again. Sometimes bending one or the other of your knees will do it. Both knees are gently bent through most of the exercise anyhow and thus in flexible readiness to assist with any correction that may be called for.

Western science provides a most interesting parallel to this ancient Tai Chi principle of being a marionette in movement. After 1900 the American George E. Coghill began the first systematic observation of embryonic behavior. The most suitable subject for such investigation, it turned out, was a kind of salamander. After an exhaustive study of its earliest stages of development Coghill discovered that all activity of this animal originates in the musculature of its head and then flashes tailward. In other words from the very start there is a dominance of the trunk over the limbs. Even after the animal grows and the limbs become more independent, they are still part of the "total pattern," this trunk dominance which Coghill found always to be the basic thing in the creature's movements.

Coghill was certain, and research now confirms, that much the same is true of human embryonic behavior. He believed however that our "total pattern" or the marionette-principle in us is corrupted by the habits of civilization, such as sitting upon chairs instead of squatting or sitting upon the ground.

Your Body Becomes Efficient

The grace and naturalness which Tai Chi imparts to you will be highly noticeable. The whole time you practice it your spine is straightened out. And this permits a release for all the organs of your body, so that they may function at top efficiency. Your trunk is never collapsed, your torso does not settle in on itself. Among other health benefits you will find an increase in endurance.

As you continue to practice there takes place a strengthening of your various leg muscles, and you gain a firmer back. This is because you are holding yourself up by the use of your own muscles rather than simply holding the body weight in balance. (The latter involves mostly a pull on the ligaments.) And the careful placement of your weight upon a single foot necessary before the execution of each step brings about a balancing of the hips, so that the back does not get hollow. The constant shifting of weight from leg to leg throughout the exercise strengthens the muscles in the buttocks. Flabby buttocks are undesirable because these muscles should be made use of in many everyday activities, like walking.

Tai Chi Relieves Backache

Muscle retraining through exercise, as well as rest and improved posture, can relieve certain cases of low backache as well as shoulder pains and even mild cases of slipped disc. If you suffer from any such complaint, however, find out first whether your doctor considers your case one likely to be benefited by exercise.

Adapt Tai Chi
to Your Body

Tall, short, thin, fat, lanky, or padded, and whatever the proportions of your body, there is nothing to prevent you from learning this exercise, and doing it well. For as the Chinese put it, each person will inevitably find his own Tai Chi. By this is meant that you adjust the exercise to your own body as you go along.

If you have a short torso and long legs do not expect to look like someone else who is doing it with short legs and a long torso. The basic actions are the same, to be sure, but the length of steps will vary with different people, as will the degree of knee-bend, and everything else. Therefore in the instructions there is no indication that feet should be eight inches apart. Instead it says that they should be shoulder-width apart, so that each action is in relation to *your* body.

Do not be concerned if your Tai Chi is not at first as beautifully executed as you would like. Do it regularly and by degrees you will find yourself growing into the exercise. The three sections were originally devised, as has been mentioned, in such a way that each section is made easier by the completion of the one before. The plan of instruction offered in this book has also been worked out according to a gradual progress of lessons. Find your own stride, and in the order given take on each new lesson without haste when you are ready for it.

Remember, you are not in competition with anybody. You are doing Tai Chi only for yourself, for your own good—for the benefits in health, pleasure and tranquillity that will follow.

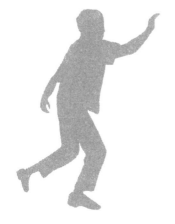

PART II

THE PRACTICE OF TAI CHI
How to do it

The Ten Basic Rules

1. Relax. Avoid any nervous or muscular tension. Relax facial muscles as well, and avoid any conscious facial expression. The result will be a look of serenity.

2. Empty your mind of thought and allow it to become wholly concerned with and aware of each movement of the body.

3. Perform the actions as slowly as possible.

4. Keep the same tempo throughout. Some actions lend themselves to a faster tempo, but avoid any such temptation to hurry.

5. Breathe easily and naturally through the nose.

6. Every action should be comfortable. If it is not comfortable, it is not correct.

7. Never push any action to the utmost. Never step as far as possible, or push arms as far as possible. Always reserve the end of the action to become the beginning of the next one.

8. Every action should be performed with careful deliberateness. Nothing is unimportant. Perform each action as though for the first time.

9. No conscious strength or force should ever be exerted. All motions should be soft and gentle.

10. Action is continuous from the beginning of Tai Chi to the end of Tai Chi. Never stop an action. Never be completely still.

A Way to Begin

If possible, have someone read aloud the instructions. (The indented notes following the instructions offer commentary and further detail, and need not be read while learning.) Follow the instructions slowly until you have an idea of what the action is. Then do it and have someone correct you from the book. Do not stop until you can do the action from memory. You can then refer back to the book during your own practice sessions. But for the first reading of any lesson, it is a good idea to have an assistant. You might try working with someone else or with a group regularly so that you can correct each other.

Tai Chi, however, should never be thought of as a performance or an exhibition. You do it for yourself only. Others may be helpful while you are learning, but your daily practice should be alone or with someone else who is practicing seriously.

Loosen your clothes before beginning to allow as much freedom as possible. Unbutton your shirt collar and open your belt. Women will not be able to do Tai Chi in high heels: any kind of slipper or low-heel shoe is satisfactory.

In practicing never do over and over again an isolated action. Do what comes before and then the action and then what comes after. Avoid exhaustion this way. In following these instructions, you will find that a continuous movement is less tiring than stopping and constantly repeating a segment.

Continued practice will make breathing deeper and more regular. Greater development in this must be left for advanced students, but beginners will in time find their own natural places for breathing, such as: inhale when pulling in, and exhale when pushing out.

Although one must strive toward perfection, one must not give up for lack of it. Do as well as possible and realize that one is always learning refinements.

Six Helpful Hints

1. The knee of the forward leg should never bend forward so deeply that it goes beyond the toe of the foot.

2. The head, neck and spine must always be in a line, with back and torso straight but not rigid. (No military posture!) Head and eye movements are as important as any other movements and should not be neglected.

3. Feet should be placed slowly and deliberately in position, feet coming down heel first on forward movements and toe first on backward steps, except where specially noted to the contrary.

4. Never lift one foot to take a step until the balance has been firmly established on the other foot.

5. Weight should always be on one foot, never on both, except at the beginning of Section One, Section Two and Section Three and at the end of the complete cycle of exercises. With few exceptions both legs are bent throughout.

6. Arm movements are usually circular, describing or completing a circle. Usually the hand which has been lower rises and the upper hand descends.

Section One

Lesson One:

❧   1. **Beginning of Tai Chi.** Face north, with feet parallel, toes pointed straight ahead, feet about shoulder-width apart, arms hanging loosely at sides, palms naturally curved and facing back. Arms rise slowly forward to about shoulder height. By drawing elbows down toward sides, draw hands in toward chest, palms curved and facing slightly downward, fingers still pointing north. As hands lower toward knees, body lowers slowly, knees bending, torso held straight. The body is in a position as though just about to sit.

NOTE:

The directions north, south, etc., are used only for convenience in describing the actions. Whichever direction you are facing when you start will be assumed to be north. Leave most room to your left.

Before beginning, relax as completely as possible, allowing the arms to hang at the sides naturally. Breathe normally. When the arms begin to rise, it should be without effort, as though they were rising to the surface of water. When they lower, it should be without force or effort, like leaves falling from a tree. As hands draw in toward chest, wrists are not bent.

✿   ✿   ✿

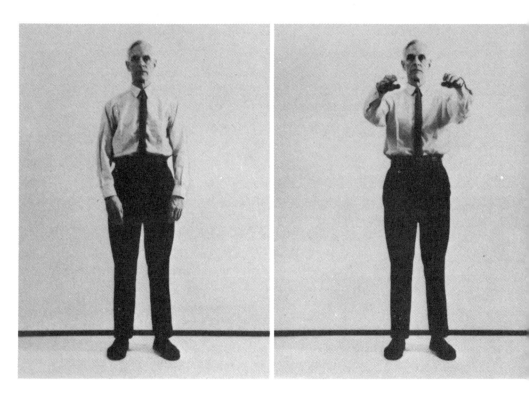

Form 1: *Beginning of Tai Chi*   **Form 1 (plate 2)**

Lesson Two:

2. **Grasp Bird's Tail Right.** With weight on left foot, right foot turns on heel to east. As hands move to hold a big ball close to the abdomen, left hand over ball, right hand beneath, body turns to east. Right foot steps east, right knee bending, weight shifting to right foot, as right hand rises chin-high over right knee, palm facing in, and left hand descends to side of left leg, palm facing back. Left leg is slightly bent.

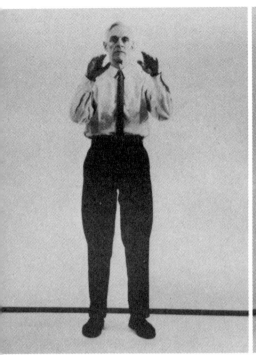 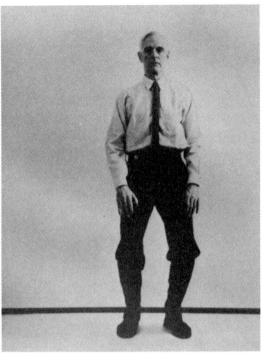

Form 1 (plate 3)   Form 1 (plate 4)

NOTE:

Hands and arms move at the same time as body and feet. All actions are continuous. Hands are curved naturally. When hands move to hold ball, the left hand is curved downward to fit the top of a ball and the right hand is curved up to hold the bottom of a ball. When the right leg bends and weight shifts to right foot, the right knee must not extend beyond the right toe. The torso must be kept upright. The eyes look at the raised right hand.

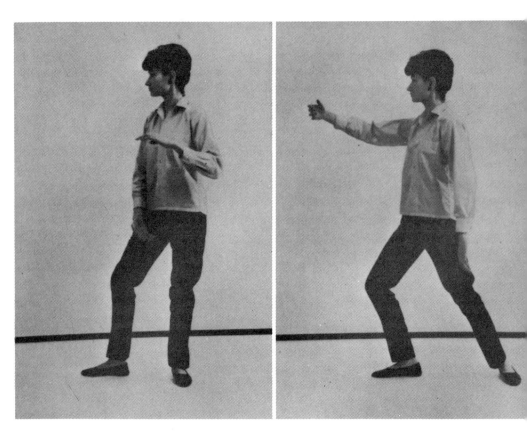

Form 2: *Grasp Bird's Tail Right*   **Form 2 (plate 2)**

3. Grasp Bird's Tail Left. Left hand moves under right elbow, palm facing up, and right arm turns north, right palm down. Left foot steps north, left heel at right angle to right heel, left knee bending, and body turns to north. As weight shifts to left foot, right hand descends to the side of right leg, palm facing back, and left hand rises chin-high over left knee, palm facing in.

NOTE:

This action is similar to No. 2. It is important to face the torso directly north. Do not tip forward, but keep torso upright. The eyes look at raised left hand.

❀   ❀   ❀

Form 3: *Grasp Bird's Tail Left*   **Form 3 (plate 2)**

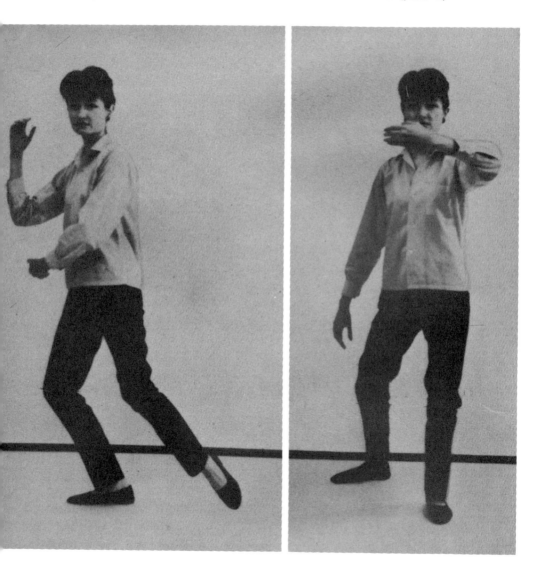

Lesson Three:

4. Push Up. Weight shifts to right foot as left foot turns on heel to east, body turning east at the same time. Hands form small ball in front of body, waist-high, left hand on top. Weight shifts to left foot and right foot steps southeast as hands push ball slanting upward to the southeast, right knee bending and weight shifting to right foot. Left leg is also slightly bent. As right foot steps, body also turns to southeast.

NOTE:

Again, it is important to avoid tipping body forward. Body should face solidly toward southeast as hands push up. Avoid leading with right shoulder.

Form 4: *Push Up*　　　　　　　　**Form 4 (plate 2)**

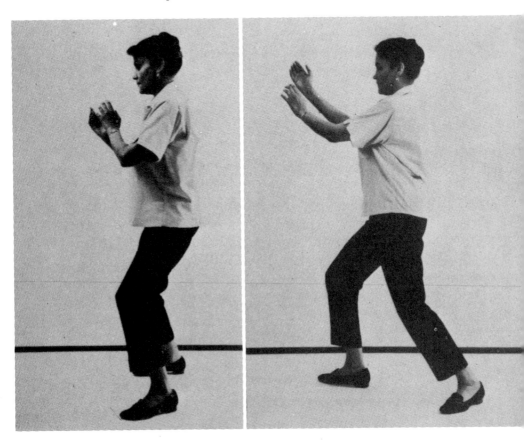

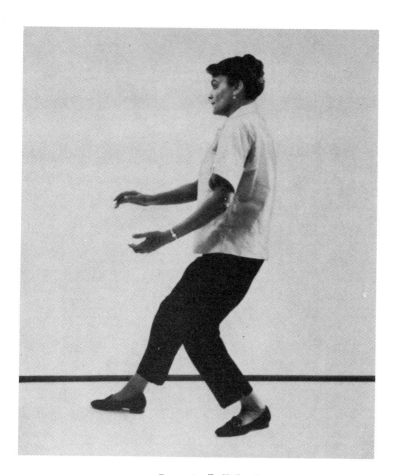

Form 5: *Pull Back*

5. Pull Back. Hands reverse to right over left, and arms draw down and back toward left side, as body pulls back and weight shifts to left foot.

NOTE:

As hands reverse, the back of the right hand is before the face. Hands are still in "ball-holding" position. Then as hands pull back, the left palm faces up and the right palm down. As hands draw further down, they close almost to fists, opening again as they push forward in No. 6.

❀   ❀   ❀

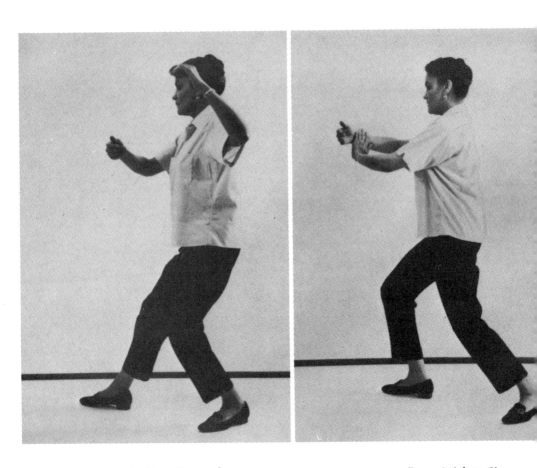

Form 6: *Press Forward*

Form 6 (plate 2)

Lesson Four:

6. Press Forward. Left hand circles back and comes forward to rest on right wrist, pushing wrist forward at heart level, as weight shifts to right foot, right knee bending. The right palm faces in.

NOTE:

The left hand meets the right wrist about ten inches in front of the chest. The fingers of the left hand rest on the right wrist.

7. Separate Hands and Push. Hands separate outward, left passing over right. Hands pull back toward chest by dropping elbows, palms facing out, as weight shifts to left foot. Hands push forward and slightly downward, as weight shifts to right foot, right knee bending.

Form 7: *Separate Hands and Push*   **Form 7 (plate 2)**

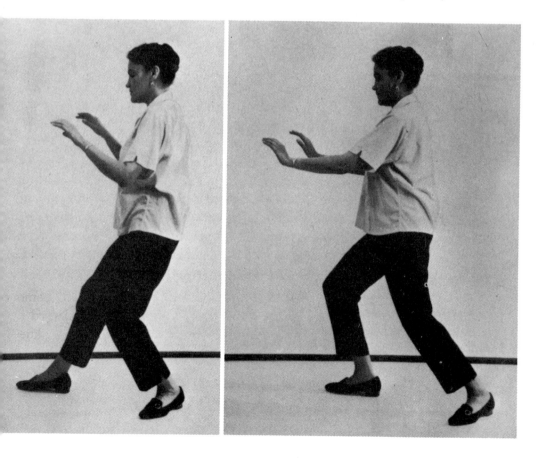

NOTE:

As hands separate, arms are about shoulder-width apart. As hands push forward and downward, it should *feel* as though the body pushes. However, there should be no force or effort in the push. The movement must be as gentle as all the other movements, but you should think of pushing.

❀   ❀   ❀

Lesson Five:

8. Turn Body to Single Whip. Head turns north. Body pulls back, weight shifting to left foot, as right foot turns leftward on heel to northwest. Body turns at same time, arms still held out at shoulder height and shoulder-width apart. Weight shifts to right foot as arms turn northwest and draw in, right hand drawing in toward chest and then out to northeast over right leg, fingers pinched together, pointing down, right elbow bent. Left hand curves inward toward waist, then upward toward right side of chest and then stretches southwest, left palm turning out and down, as left foot turns and steps southwest. Left knee bends as weight shifts to left foot.

NOTE:

This is probably the most difficult action to perfect. The body and arms begin to turn as the right foot begins to turn. By the time the right foot is in position (pointing northwest) the arms will be stretched out at shoulder level also pointing northwest. Before the left foot steps, the arms begin to draw in toward the body, which is now facing north. The left hand swings down toward the waist and the right hand circles in at chest height. The right hand begins to form the pinched fist as it comes in toward the chest. It then stretches out to the northeast at shoulder height, with the elbow bent. At this point, the left hand has come up before the right side of the chest, palm facing in. The body turns, the left hand extends to the southwest at shoulder height, and the left foot steps to the southwest, all at the same time. The left arm is not straight but slightly curved. The left hand turns out and down so that the palm faces down. The body faces southwest. The right hand now points north as a result of the body's turning to the southwest.

The right foot turns slightly to adjust the balance of the body as the body turns to the southwest, right foot turning to slightly west of northwest.

Practice this action very carefully. It is repeated more often than any other in the entire series of 108. Do not tip the torso forward at any point.

❖　❖　❖

Form 8: *Turn Body to Single Whip*

Form 8 (plate 2)

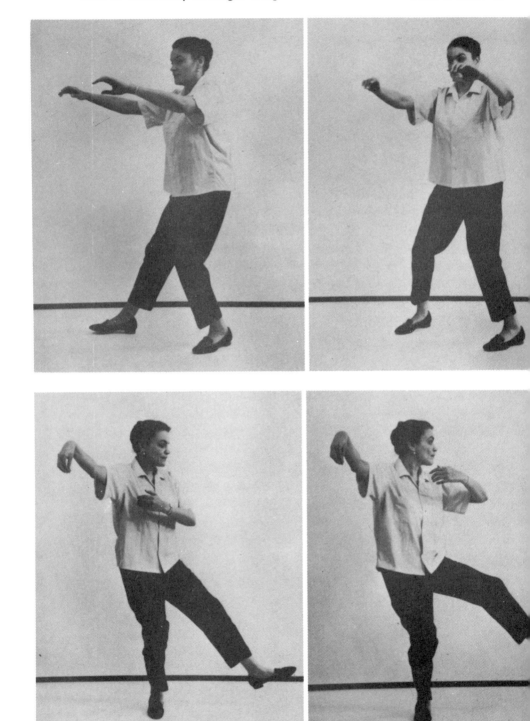

Form 8 (plate 5)   Form 8 (plate 6)

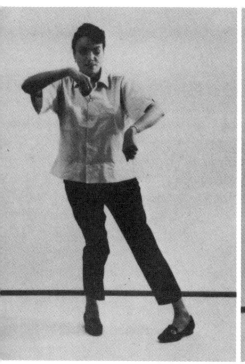

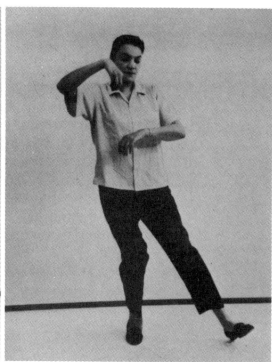

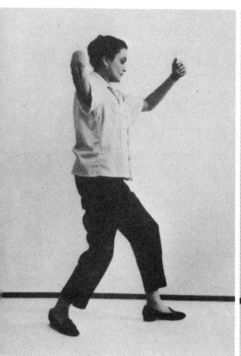

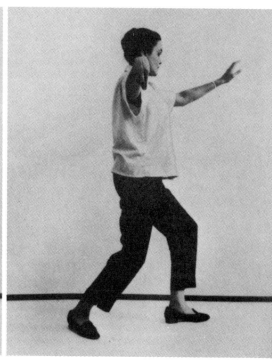

Form 8 (plate 7)

Form 8 (plate 8)

Lesson Six:

9. Raise Hands and Step Up. Weight shifts to right foot. Left foot turns on heel slightly to west, weight shifting to left foot as right foot turns on sole of foot to north, heel raised. Palms open and arms open wide. Right foot steps north, heel touching floor, toe raised, as arms close in, left hand coming to a point between right wrist and elbow, not quite touching right arm. Left palm faces right and right palm faces left. Arms pull back and down toward left side, and right foot draws back to left foot, right toe only touching floor, weight remaining on left foot. Left hand continues backward, circling forward to rest left palm on inside of right arm between wrist and elbow, closer to wrist. Right foot steps slightly to the left of north, weight shifting to right foot and right knee bending as left hand pushes right arm to north, right elbow leading.

NOTE:

Before the right foot steps north it is essential to establish the weight firmly on the left foot, so that the right foot can move *slowly* into position. As the arms close in, they assume a position similar to "Play Guitar" in No. 12. The arms are stretched out in front of the body, slightly curved, pointing north. As arms pull back and right foot steps back, the entire body lifts up. This is one of the few actions in which the leg bearing the weight is not bent.

✽   ✽   ✽

Form 9: *Raise Hands and Step Up*　　　　　　　　**Form 9 (plate 2)**

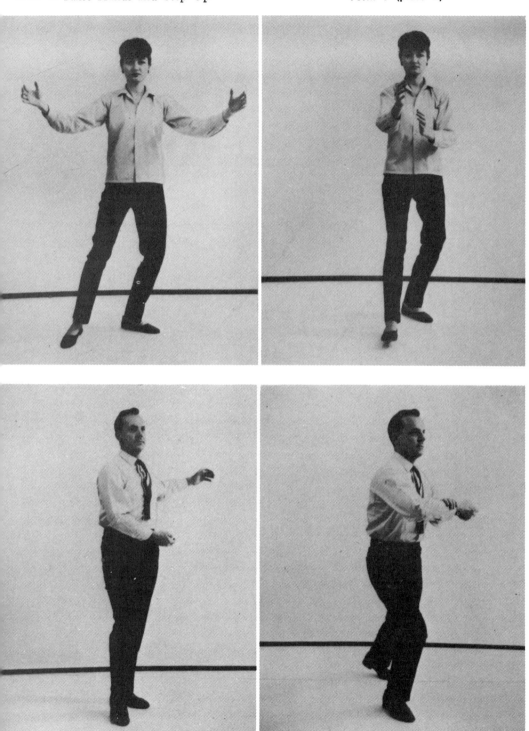

Form 9 (plate 3)　　　　　　　　**Form 9 (plate 4)**

10. Stork Spreads Wings. Weight is on right foot, right knee bent. Body turns west as right foot turns on sole to northwest and left foot turns on sole to west. Left foot steps southwest with heel raised, toe only touching floor. Right hand rises before face, palm down, fingers pointing south, as left hand lowers to left side, palm facing back. Weight remains on right foot, right knee bent.

NOTE:
> In this position both legs are bent and the pelvis is tucked under, giving a concave appearance to the body.

❀   ❀   ❀

Form 10:
Stork Spreads Wings

Lesson Eight:

Review. In the first seven lessons all the basic principles of Tai Chi have been demonstrated. Read again the Ten Basic Rules on page 67 and test yourself to be sure you are observing all of them in your practice. Do not proceed to Lesson Nine until you are absolutely certain that you are practicing the first ten actions correctly.

Pay special attention to your head, neck and spine alignment. The Tai Chi trunk is a straight one. Especially in Push Up and the following actions (Nos. 4 through 7), beginners have a tendency to tip forward from the hips in the direction of the hands. Check your position in front of a mirror. Compare with photographs. If you are tipping forward, bend the left leg more deeply and you will see at once that the deeper bend will correct the position of the trunk, lowering your body and straightening your back.

Read again the instructions for each action. Be sure that your arm and leg movements are synchronized and coordinated.

Check to see whether there is any tenseness in your body or your face. In the beginning you may find that concentration on mastering the actions will cause tension in the face muscles or clenching of teeth or lips. Practice each lesson until you have learned the movements so thoroughly that this type of extreme concentration can be eliminated. The motions should flow easily and comfortably.

Be sure that your weight shifts completely from foot to foot as indicated in the instructions. Weight shifting is one of the most important aspects of Tai Chi, and failure to shift weight will make the practice much less beneficial.

❋ ❋ ❋

Lesson Nine:

11. Brush Knee and Twist Left. Right hand circles down to hold bottom of ball at right side, left hand coming up to hold top of ball. Left foot steps southwest as left hand, palm down, descends to brush past left knee. Right hand circles back and pushes forward, palm down, to southwest at eye level, weight shifting to left foot, left knee bending, as body turns to the southwest. Right leg is slightly bent.

NOTE:

This is one of the basic, often repeated actions. Particular attention should be given to keeping the torso straight and not tipping forward from the waist. Right leg should be bent enough to avoid tipping forward.

As the right hand circles back and then pushes forward it comes forward past the right ear, not higher. The circling motion is from the shoulder, not the elbow.

All Brush Knee and Twist actions face a "corner," in this case southwest. In later repeats of this movement the direction will be to the northwest, southeast, and southwest.

❋ ❋ ❋

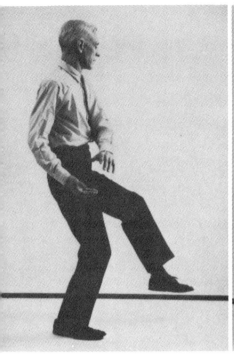

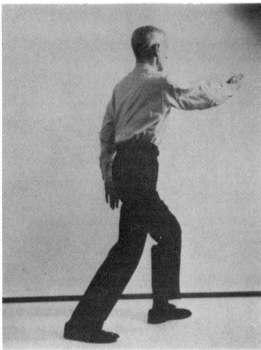

Form 11: *Brush Knee and Twist Left*   **Form 11 (plate 2)**

Lesson Ten:

12.   **Play Guitar.** Right foot takes small step up but not coming up as far as left foot. Weight shifts to right foot, right knee bending. Left foot steps forward, heel touching floor, toe slightly raised. Left arm comes up and forward over left foot, and right arm comes down to a point between left elbow and wrist, but not touching left arm. The right palm faces the inside of the left forearm, and left palm faces north. The body faces west.

NOTE:

This is similar to No. 9, except that the left arm is leading. All "Play Guitar" actions face directly west.

❋   ❋   ❋

Form 12: *Play Guitar*

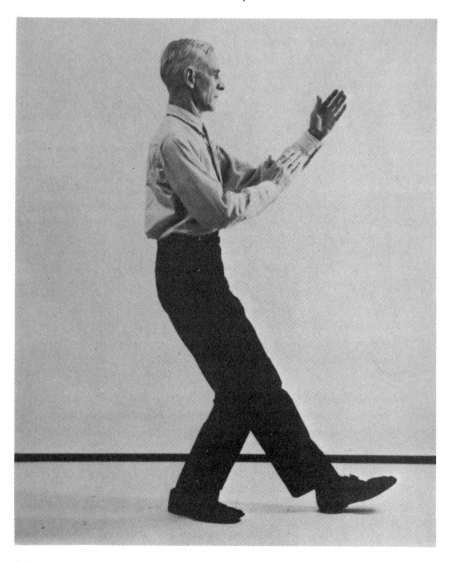

Lesson Eleven:

13. **Brush Knee and Twist Left.** Hands enclose ball at right hip, left hand on top. Left foot steps southwest, weight shifting to left foot, left knee bending, and hands brush and push as in No. 11.

14. **Brush Knee and Twist Right.** Weight shifts back to right foot, as left foot turns on heel very slightly to the left. Hands enclose ball at left hip, right hand on top. Weight shifts to left foot, left knee bending. Right foot takes large step to the northwest, weight shifting to right foot, right knee bending, as right hand, palm down,

Form 14: *Brush Knee and Twist Right*   **Form 14 (plate 2)**

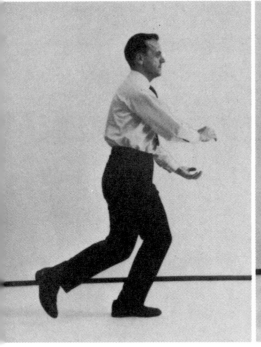
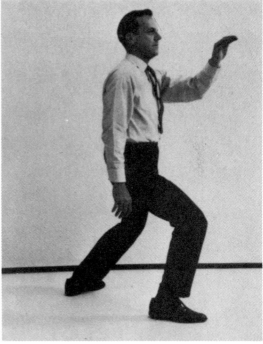

descends and brushes past right knee, and left hand circles back and pushes forward to the northwest over right knee, palm down, body turning at the same time to the northwest.

NOTE:

The reason that the left foot turns very slightly to the left is to make certain that the body is in balance when the right foot steps forward.

15. Brush Knee and Twist Left. Weight shifts to left foot as right foot turns on heel very slightly to the right. Hands enclose ball at right hip, left hand on top. Weight shifts to right foot, right knee bending, and left foot takes large step to the southwest, weight shifting to left foot, left knee bending, as hands brush and push as in No. 11.

16. Play Guitar. The same action as No. 12.

17. Brush Knee and Twist Left. The same action as No. 13.

❁   ❁   ❁

Lesson Twelve:

18. Strike Fist to Right. Right hand forms loose fist. Right arm circles to right, outward and down, fist coming close to abdomen. Right arm continues circling clockwise to left, up in front of face and out to the right (north), as though chopping an opponent on the top of the head. Weight is still on the left foot.

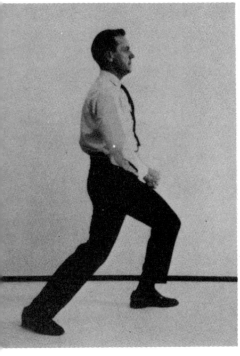 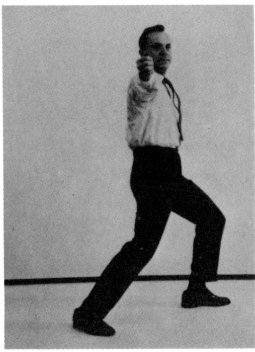

Form 18: *Strike Fist to Right*   **Form 18 (plate 2)**

NOTE:

As the right arm circles down to abdomen, the head turns to the north. The eyes are then directed at the chopping fist. The fist is held upright with the back of the palm facing east.

✻   ✻   ✻

Lesson Thirteen:

19. Step Forward and Punch. Weight shifts to right foot as left toe turns slightly to the left. Weight shifts to left foot, left knee bending, and right foot takes large step to the northwest, weight shifting to right foot, right knee bending as right arm continues to circle down, fist coming up in front of body. Right arm, elbow bent, then draws back along right side, waist-high, as left arm swings up before chest, left palm facing in. Left foot takes large step to the southwest, weight shifting to left foot, left knee bending, as right arm curves up, straightening out at waist level, right fist punching *slowly* to the west. Left hand meets and rests on inside of right elbow.

NOTE:

The "punching fist" is formed with the middle knuckle protruding slightly beyond the knuckles of the other three fingers. Thumb is on top of fist, bending down. Here the palm of the fist faces south.

✿   ✿   ✿

Form 19: *Step Forward and Punch*

Form 19 (plate 2)

Form 19 (plate 3)

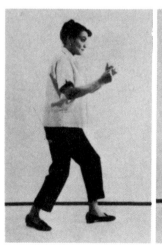
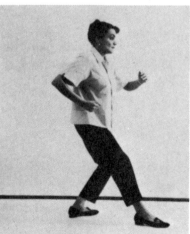
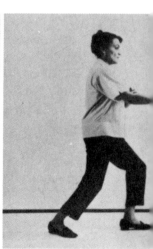

Lesson Fourteen:

20. Cross Hands. Weight shifts to right foot and body draws back. Left palm slides below right elbow. Right arm draws back, as left hand moves forward, palm up, under right arm. Right fist loosens to open palm and both arms pull back and then push forward to west, palms facing out, as weight shifts to left foot, left knee bending. Hands move upward to cross over head, left wrist over right, palms still facing out, as body turns to north. Weight shifts to right foot and left foot turns on heel to the north as arms make big descending circle outward. Weight shifts to left foot as right foot turns on heel to the north. Hands come up in front of chest, palms facing in, right wrist crossed over left, as right foot steps back even with left

Form 20: *Cross Hands*   **Form 20 (plate 2)**

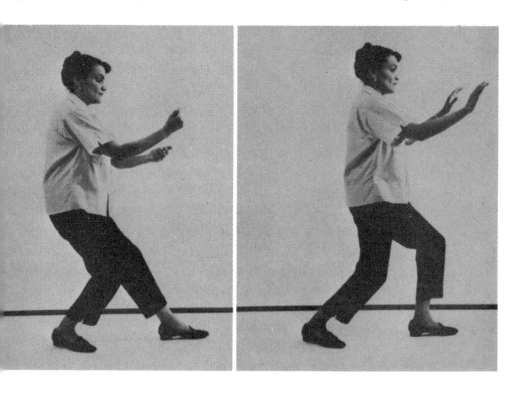

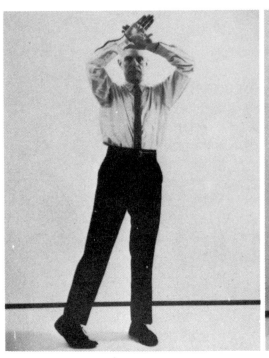
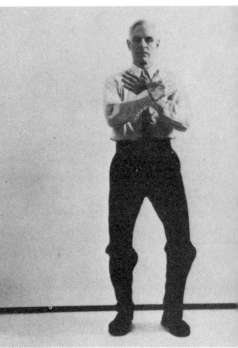

Form 20 (plate 3)   Form 20 (plate 4)

foot, shoulder-width apart. Weight is now evenly distributed on both feet, both knees bent. Hands separate and lower toward knees.

NOTE:

If Tai Chi is to be continued into Section Two, the action of No. 20 ends here. If Tai Chi is not to be continued, Section One ends here as follows:

Arms rise to shoulder level, stretching out in front of body. As knees straighten and body rises to standing position, arms are loosely curved and fingers point north, palms facing down. Elbows drop as hands draw back toward body. Arms slowly lower to starting position.

✿   ✿   ✿

Lesson Fifteen:

Review. Before proceeding to the next lesson which will take you into Section Two of Tai Chi, it would be well at this point to spend some time in careful observation and correction of your form or manner of practicing. You should now review all the Ten Basic Rules and test each of your actions against these rules. If, for example, on Single Whip you are allowing the torso to tip forward during the turn, or keeping the weight on both feet at once, without the necessary shift in weight from one foot to the other, now is the time to make these corrections and practice the movements with the corrections before moving on to Section Two.

Sections Two and Three contain repeats of every action which you have now learned with the single exception of the widening of the arms after Single Whip. It is therefore very important to have a correct way of doing these basic actions.

Check your head position in each action. Your eyes must also be moving according to the instructions. Your head should be upright on your neck and never tipped. You should feel as though there were a plumb line from the top of your head to the base of your spine.

Check your arm movements. Your arms should always be gently curved and should move freely from the shoulder. The fingers are never straight, but always loosely and naturally curved.

Check your shoulder positions. The shoulders must stay in line with the torso. The shoulders never turn or twist without taking the torso with them. For example, in Push Up, Pull Back, Press Forward, Separate Hands and Push (Nos. 4 through 7), the torso should face squarely to the southeast. As the left arm circles back in order to come forward and press the right wrist, the shoulders should not turn to the left. The body remains facing southeast and the arms swing back, independently, from the shoulder. In Brush Knee actions the torso should face the same direction as the forward hand and the shoulders do not twist as the arm circles back or pushes forward.

Check your leg positions. Observe your knee-bends in all actions. In Push Up, Pull Back, Press Forward, Separate Hands and Push, be sure that the left leg is bent deeply enough to allow the spine and torso to be upright.

Check your leg positions. Observe your knee-bends in carefully regarding the placement of the feet. These have been established to provide correct balance and weight distribution.

Be sure that you are practicing correctly. Incorrect practice establishes habits which are harder to correct later.

When you find that you have followed the instructions and can consistently practice Section One without violating any of the Ten Basic Rules, you are ready to go on to Section Two.

Section Two

Lesson One:

❦ **21. Carry Tiger to Mountain.**
From position just before
"NOTE" *(page 96)*: weight shifts
to left foot. Right hand brushes past right leg, palm down,
as right foot takes a very wide step to the southeast, weight
shifting to right foot, right knee bending. Left arm circles
back and then forward to the southeast about eye level,
open palm facing south, as left foot turns on sole to east.

Form 21: *Carry Tiger to Mountain*   **Form 21 (plate 2)**

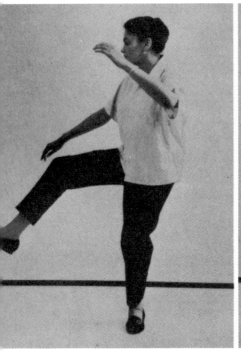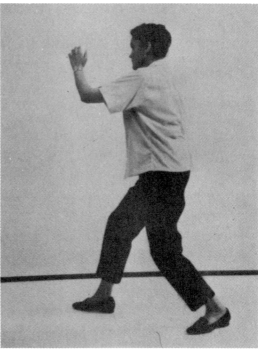

NOTE:

In this action balance is very important because the tendency is to tip the body as the right foot steps. To avoid this, be sure of firm balance on the left foot before stepping with the right foot. The left foot turns to adjust to the new balance of weight on the right foot. The right arm moves as the right foot steps, and the left arm moves as the left foot turns.

22. Push Up, Pull Back, Press Forward, Separate Hands and Push. Both hands draw back to left hip, holding ball, right hand on top, as weight shifts to left foot. Weight shifts to right foot as hands push up as in No. 4. Forms No. 5, No. 6, and No. 7 are repeated.

Form 23: *Turn Body to Single Whip*   **Form 23 (plate 2)**   **Form 23 (plate**

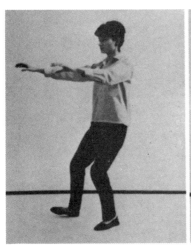 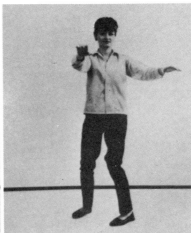 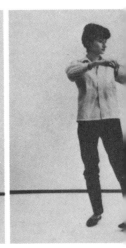

23. Turn Body to Single Whip. The same action as No. 8, except that in this instance the left foot, left arm, and body face directly to the west instead of to the southwest.

      ✿   ✿   ✿

Lesson Two:

24. Fist Under Elbow. Weight shifts to right foot and left foot takes a small step to the southwest. Right hand drops toward right side, as left arm pushes out and down toward the left, palm facing out, as weight shifts to left foot. Right foot steps forward, as right hand comes up in front of left side of chest, palm facing in, and left

Form 23 (plate 4)   **Form 23 (plate 5)**   **Form 23 (plate 6)**

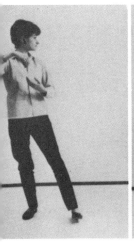
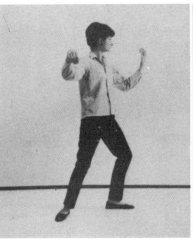
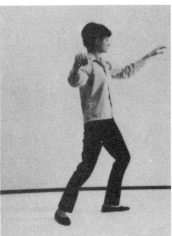

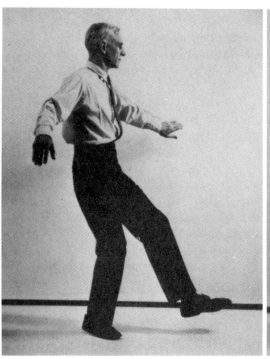 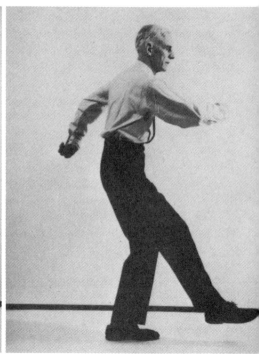

Form 24: *Fist Under Elbow*   **Form 24 (plate 2)**

hand continues circling back and then forward under left
armpit, coming up inside right arm, fingers pointing
upward, palm facing in. Weight shifts to right foot and
left foot steps forward with only heel touching floor, as
left hand continues up inside right arm, left palm turning
outward and downward as right hand forms fist under left
elbow. The fist is upright, palm facing south.

NOTE:

The synchronization of movement is important in this
action. It may be helpful in the beginning to think
of it in three counts. Count *one* as left foot steps and
left hand pushes out and right arm drops. Count *two*

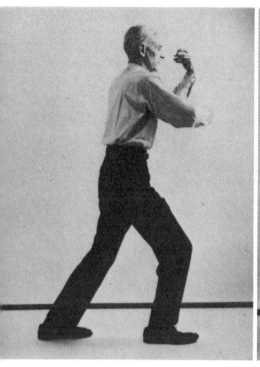 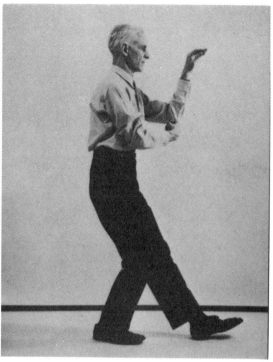

Form 24 (plate 3)   Form 24 (plate 4)

as right foot steps, right arm comes forward before
chest and left arm begins to curve up from behind.
Count *three* as left foot steps, left hand comes forward and right hand forms fist under elbow.

❖   ❖   ❖

Lesson Three:

25. Step Back and Repulse Monkey. Right fist
loosens to open palm, facing up, and right arm drops down

and back. Left foot steps back, weight shifting to left foot, as left hand, palm up, sinks to left hip and continues to circle back; at the same time, right arm continues to circle back, around, and forward, palm facing out, as though pushing. Right foot steps back, weight shifting to right foot, as right hand, palm up, sinks to right hip and circles back, and left hand circles down, back, up and pushes forward, palm out. Repeat action with left foot stepping back, then right foot, then left foot, making five steps back in all, with accompanying arm movements.

NOTE:

Again, synchronization is important. Left foot and left arm move backwards together, and right foot and right arm move backwards together. Both legs are

Form 25: *Step Back and*
Repulse Monkey

Form 25 (plate 2)

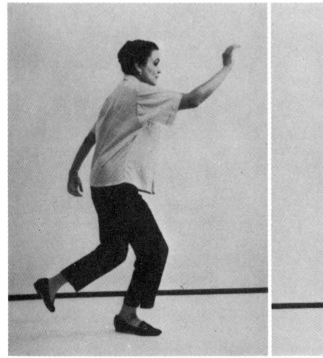
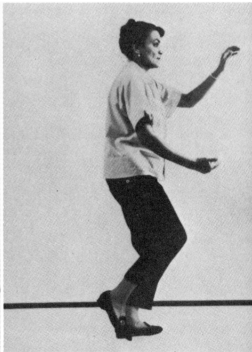

bent at all times and the torso is slightly concave, although upright. As the right foot and right arm are moving back and the left hand pushing forward, the hands enclose a ball in passing, left hand on top. As each foot steps back it must step directly back, toes still pointing west. Feet should step back shoulder-width apart and parallel to each other.

✿   ✿   ✿

Lesson Four:

26.   Slanting Flying. Weight is on the left foot. Right arm circles down and outward and left arm circles back

Form 25 (plate 3)   **Form 25 (plate 4)**

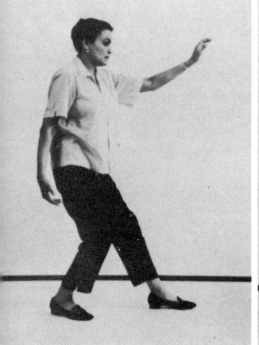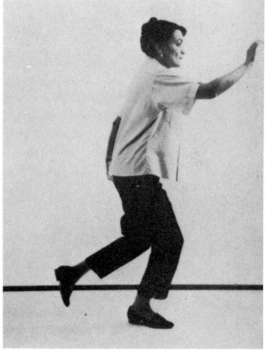

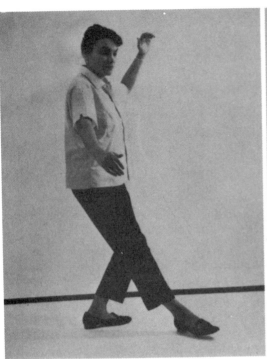

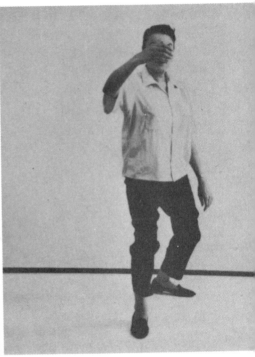

Form 26: *Slanting Flying*

Form 26 (plate 2)

and up. (Hands and arms circle clockwise, in very large circle, palms facing each other.) Hands form ball close to body at waist level, left hand on top, as body turns to face north, right foot turning slightly on heel to the northwest with toe lifted. Right foot steps north, weight shifting to right foot, right knee bending, and right hand rises over right knee about chin-high, palm facing in, as left hand descends along left leg, palm facing back.

NOTE:

Body is quite concave as arms make big clockwise circle. It is necessary to establish the weight firmly on the left foot before stepping north with right foot.

27. Raise Hands and Step Up. The same action as No. 9, starting at point where arms pull back and down.

28. Stork Spreads Wings. The same action as No. 10.

29. Brush Knee and Twist Left. The same action as No. 11.

❁   ❁   ❁

Lesson Five:

30. Needle at Sea Bottom. Weight is on left foot. Right foot takes a small step forward, but not passing left foot. Weight shifts to right foot, as left foot takes a small step forward with only toe touching floor. Left hand touches inside of right elbow as body lowers and bends forward from waist, knees bent. Right hand points down near inside of left foot. Weight remains on right foot.

NOTE:

> Although the torso bends forward from the waist, the body is lowered as much by the bending of the legs as by tipping forward. The right leg is rather deeply bent. When the right hand points down, the palm faces south, with index and second fingers pointed down, third and fourth fingers slightly bent inward, and thumb pointing down. Head is upright, not bent down, and eyes are looking straight ahead.

❁   ❁   ❁

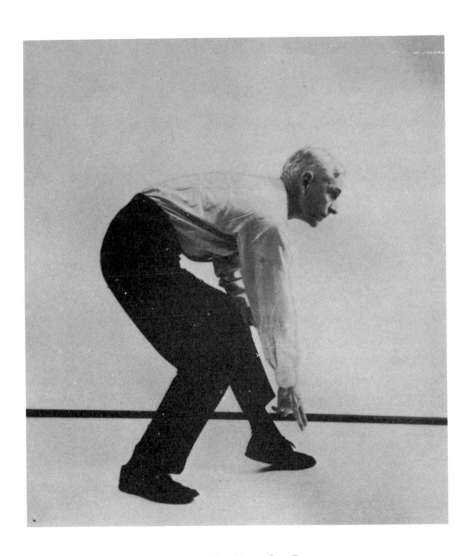

Form 30: *Needle at Sea Bottom*

Lesson Six:

31. Raise Arms Like Fan. Body straightens up, hands pulling back toward chest, palms out, elbows lowering. Left foot steps slightly forward, weight shifting to left foot, left knee bending, as arms push forward in front of face, palms facing out, left hand slightly higher than right.

NOTE:

The palms should be a little more than shoulder-width apart, but not too wide. The left hand is slightly above face level. The hands are loosely curved, with fingers slightly spread.

Form 31: *Raise Arms Like Fan*

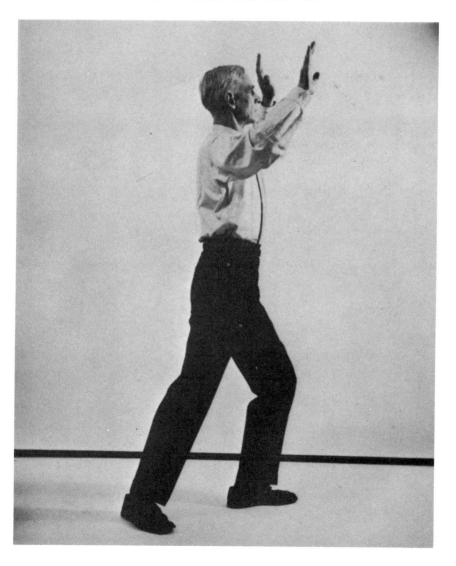

32. Turn Body and Strike Fist Back. Right hand forms fist and lowers to abdomen as left hand lowers to left side, palm back. Head and body turn to face north. Both feet turn north. Head turns to east as right fist comes up in front of body, circling clockwise up and out to the right (east).

NOTE:

This is a normal fist without protruding knuckle. As it strikes out to the east, the fist is upright with thumb on top, palm of fist facing north.

✿　✿　✿

Form 32: *Turn Body and*
Strike Fist Back

Form 32 (plate 2)

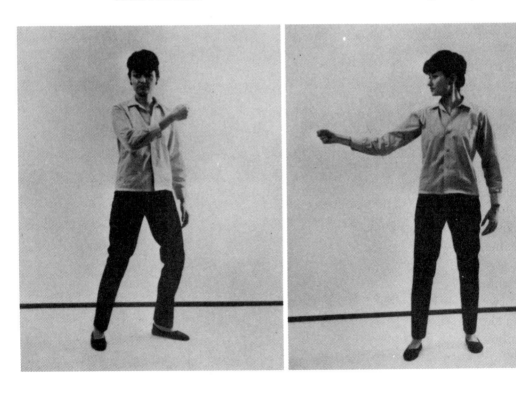

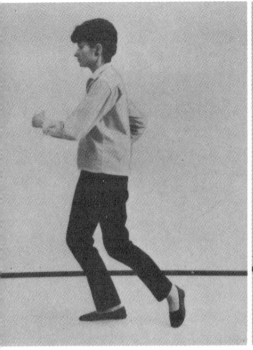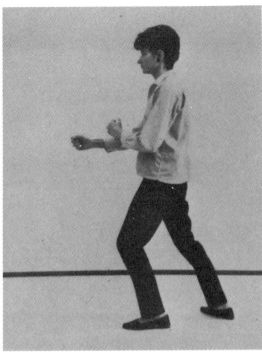

Form 33: *Step Forward and Punch*

Lesson Seven:

33. **Step Forward and Punch.** With weight on left foot, right foot steps southeast, weight shifting to right foot, right knee bending. Right arm continues circling down, with fist coming up in front of chest, as left arm comes forward in front of chest, palm facing in. Right arm draws back at waist level, right elbow extending backward behind body. Left foot steps east and right arm comes forward, curving under, and straightens out at waist level in slow punch, left palm coming to rest on inside of right elbow.

NOTE:

>This is a "punching fist," with middle knuckle protruding. The step of the right foot is a small one, amounting to little more than lifting the foot, turning it to point southeast, and putting it down again.

34. Push Up, Pull Back, Press Forward, Separate Hands and Push. The same action as No. 22, except weight is already on left foot.

35. Turn Body to Single Whip. The same action as No. 8. To the southwest.

✿   ✿   ✿

Form 36: *Wave Hands Like Clouds*   **Form 36 (plate 2)**   **Form 36 (plate 3)**

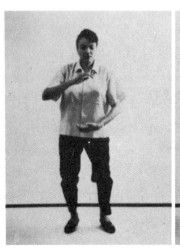 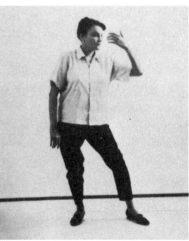 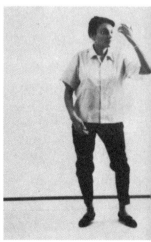

Lesson Eight:

36. Wave Hands Like Clouds. Weight shifts to right foot. Body turns north as left foot steps up, parallel to right foot, both feet pointing north, shoulder-width apart, both knees bent. Both hands move in counter-clockwise circle to form a large ball close to body, right hand on top. Weight on right foot, left foot moves sideward to left, left foot still pointing north, weight shifting to left foot as left hand comes up before face, palm facing in, right hand dropping to right side. Left hand continues counter-clockwise circle, palm turning outward as arm descends. As left hand is descending, right hand circles up clockwise in front of face, palm in, as right foot moves sideward to

Form 36 (plate 4)   **Form 36 (plate 5)**   **Form 36 (plate 6)**

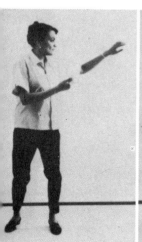
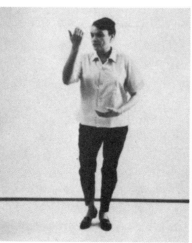
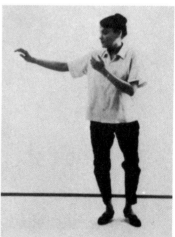

the left, right toe still pointing north. As right hand continues the circle, right palm turns outward as arm descends. In each case, the body turns from the waist in the direction of the outgoing arm. The head turns with the body and the eyes follow the outgoing hand. In each case, the weight shifts to the foot which has just moved. Repeat six times, ending with right foot stepping and right hand circling.

NOTE:

In this action both knees are bent and the body is in a sitting position during the entire action. The descending hand seems to be pushing downward and outward. The left hand makes a slightly larger circle than the right. In the beginning of this action, when the left foot steps up to join the right foot, the right foot adjusts slightly to point north.

✿ ✿ ✿

Lesson Nine:

37. Single Whip. As right hand circles up on the last "Wave Hands," it moves northeast into the Single Whip position with the fingers lightly pinched together and pointing down. The left hand, which has begun to circle up, stretches out to the southwest in the Single Whip position, as the left foot steps southwest, left knee bending and weight shifting to left foot.

NOTE:

When the body turns into the Single Whip position, the right foot, which has been pointing north, adjusts slightly to the northwest as the body turns.

38. High Pat on Horse. Right foot takes a small step forward to west, but not passing left foot. Both arms swing slightly forward and up. Right hand sinks down as weight shifts to right foot. Left foot takes very small step forward, weight shifting to left foot, left knee bending. Left hand lowers and palm turns upward, coming to rest against left thigh, while right hand circles back and then stretches out forward, as thought to pat a horse, body facing west.

NOTE:

When the hand movements are correctly coordinated with the small stepping movements, this is a very comfortable action. There is a swinging motion in the arms.

✿　✿　✿

Form 38: *High Pat on Horse*　　　　　　**Form 38 (plate 2)**

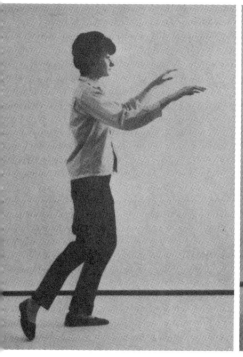 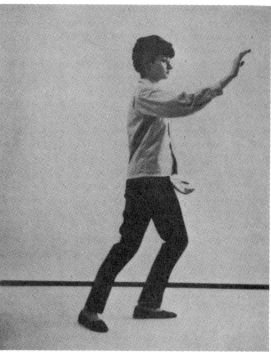

Lesson Ten:

39. Separate Right Foot. Both knees bend deeply and body bends forward. Left arm moves outward and sideward and right arm downward and outward, arms circling down, hands crossing before knees, right hand outside, palms facing in. As arms close in around knees, right foot steps up even with left foot, right toe only touching floor. Body straightens as arms open outward and upward to shoulder level and right foot comes forward and upward waist-high. Right leg then moves horizontally to the right, and then right foot returns to floor, parallel to left foot, toes pointing west, feet shoulder-width apart.

Form 39: *Separate Right Foot*   **Form 39 (plate 2)**

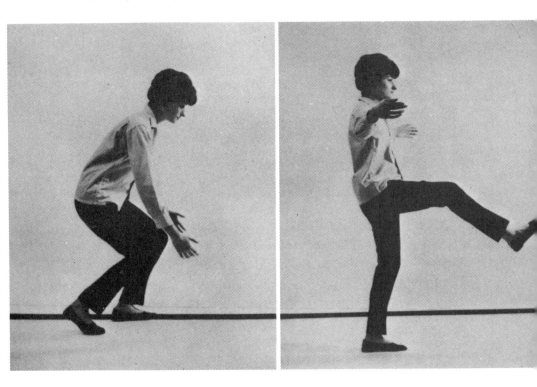

NOTE:

As body bends forward, both knees are deeply bent, lowering body. As body straightens and arms open, the right leg kicks slowly forward with foot in natural position, not tensely held upright. The right knee is slightly bent during the kick and while the right leg moves horizontally to the right. The left leg is also slightly bent.

40. Separate Left Foot. Weight shifts to right foot. Knees bend and body bends forward as left foot steps close to right foot, feet still parallel, left toe only touching floor. Arms circle down around knees as in No. 39. Body straightens as arms open outward at shoulder level and left foot kicks slowly forward waist-high and moves horizontally to the left, foot landing close to right foot, left toe only touching floor.

    ✿   ✿   ✿

Lesson Eleven:

41. Turn and Kick with Heel. Left arm swings in toward chest, right arm remaining stretched out. Body makes a half-circle turn on sole of right foot leftward to the east, left foot slightly raised from floor during turn. Arms close in front of chest, during the turn, right arm over left, both palms facing in. When the turn is completed, arms open outward at shoulder level, and left foot slowly kicks out, foot upright, as though to strike with heel.

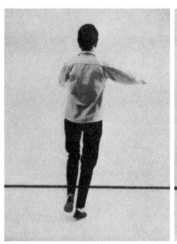 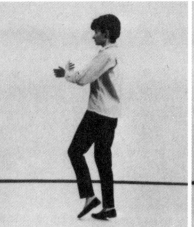 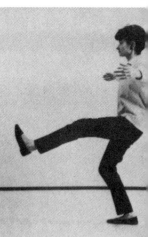

Form 41: *Turn and*   **Form 41 (plate 2)**   **Form 41 (plate 3)**
Kick with Heel

NOTE:

Weight remains on right foot throughout this action. The turn is more easily accomplished if, when you lift the right heel preparatory to turning on sole, you consciously lift the body so that the turn may be made lightly. Do not hurry, but keep the same tempo as in all other actions.

42. Brush Knee and Twist Left and Right. Hands move slightly to the right forming large ball. Without returning to the floor after the kick, left foot steps northeast, weight shifting to left foot, left knee bending, as left hand brushes past left knee and right hand pushes out over left knee as in No. 13. Then brush knee to right as in No. 14.

NOTE:

The Brush Knee and Twist steps are the same as in No. 13 and 14 except that the direction of Brush Knee Left is to the northeast and the direction of Brush Knee Right is to the southeast. At the beginning of this action, before stepping down with the left leg, the left leg bends at the knee, so that the step is a natural one, not a stiff one.

✿   ✿   ✿

Lesson Twelve:

43. Circle Hand and Punch Downward. Weight shifts to left foot. Right hand forms fist and extends forward, palm of fist down, arm circling outward and back in front of body, describing large, clockwise, horizontal circle. Meanwhile, left hand comes up in front of chest, palm facing in. (Body sits back, weight firmly on left leg, while right fist is circling.) Weight shifts to right foot and left foot steps forward to east. Body bends forward and right fist punches slowly downward toward a point in front of and to the right of left foot, left hand resting on inside of right elbow.

NOTE:

This is a "punching fist," with middle knuckle protruding. The punch down is directed as though to an opponent's instep.

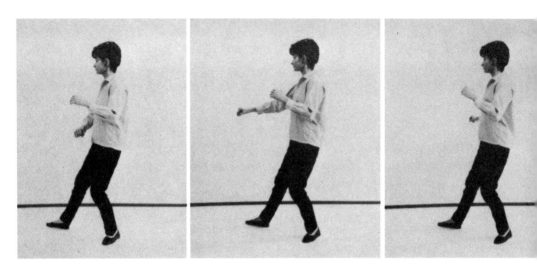

Form 43: *Circle Hand* and *Punch Downward*

Form 43 (plate 2)

Form 43 (plate 3)

44. Turn Body and Strike Fist Back. Body straightens and left arm drops to left side, palm back. Right hand, becoming normal fist, draws up to abdomen. Head and body turn to face south. Both feet turn to south and head turns to face west, as right fist comes up in front of body, circles clockwise overhead and out to the right (west). The fist remains a normal upright fist, palm facing south.

45. Step Forward and Punch. With weight on left foot, body turns to face west. Left arm comes forward before chest as right arm continues circling down, right fist coming up in front of chest. Right arm draws back at waist level, right elbow extending backward behind body, as right foot takes small step northwest, weight shifting to right foot, right knee bending. Left foot steps forward to west, weight shifting to left foot, left knee bending, as right arm comes forward, curving under, and straightens

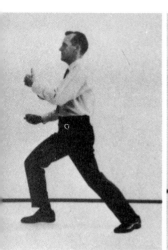 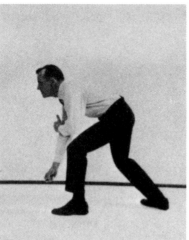

Form 43 (plate 4)   **Form 43 (plate 5)**

out at waist level in punch, left palm coming to rest at inside of right elbow. Middle knuckle of right fist protrudes.

NOTE:

Nos. 44 and 45 are similar to Nos. 32 and 33, except that the direction is different.

46. Kick Upward with Right Foot. Both knees bend deeply, weight still on left foot, as arms circle outward and downward, closing in at knees, right hand outside, both palms facing in. Right foot steps up to left foot, right toe only touching floor. Body straightens up, arms opening outward at shoulder level and right foot kicks forward, returning to floor parallel with left foot, but slightly ahead of left foot.

✿   ✿   ✿

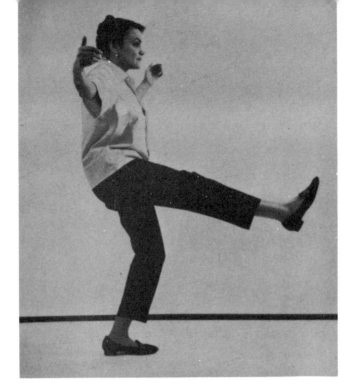

Form **46**: *Kick Upward with Right Foot*

Lesson Thirteen:

47. Hit Tiger at Left. Weight shifts to right foot. Hands pull back toward right thigh. Left foot steps south-

Form **47**: *Hit Tiger at Left*

Form **47** **(plate 2)**

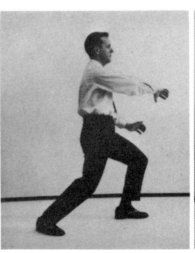
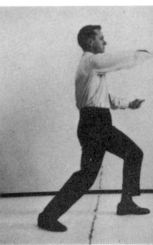

west as hands pull down toward left side, loosely open as though holding a thick pole. The right hand is higher and both palms face slantingly outward and downward. Weight shifts forward to left foot, left knee bending, as hands form fists and arms circle up from left side, over head, down toward right side, and forward and upward to the left, with left fist turned outward about one foot in front of forehead, and right fist pushing forward to southwest under left fist, but not extending beyond left fist. The direction of the fists is to the southwest, and the palm of the right fist faces left.

NOTE:

> It may be helpful to imagine that you are holding a pole, or in fact, to practice this action holding a cane or umbrella. In this way it will be easy to keep your hands the same distance apart throughout all the circling motions. If the point of the cane or umbrella is pointing down as you pull your hands down to the left side, it will have reversed so that the point is up at the end of the action.

48. Hit Tiger at Right. Weight still on left foot, right foot steps northwest, weight shifting to right foot,

Form 47 (plate 3)   **Form 47 (plate 4)**   **Form 47 (plate 5)**

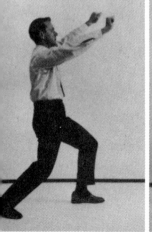
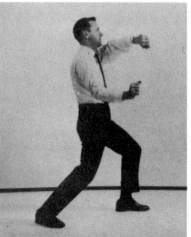
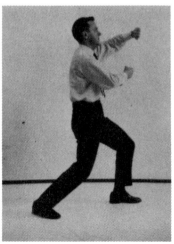

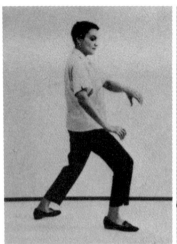 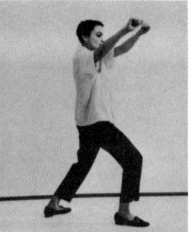 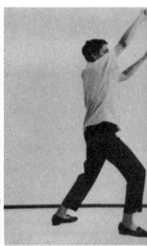

Form 48: *Hit Tiger*
at Right

Form 48 (plate 2)

Form 48 (plate 3)

right knee bending, as hands pull down to right side loosely open as in No. 47. The left hand is higher, palms facing outward and downward. Hands form fists and circle up to the right, over head, to the left and then forward to the right, right fist turning outward about one foot in front of forehead and left fist pushing under right fist, about one foot below right fist. The direction of the fists is to the northwest, and the palm of the left fist faces right.

NOTE:

In both No. 47 and No. 48 the body turns from the waist, following the motions of the circling arms. Both legs are bent.

✻　✻　✻

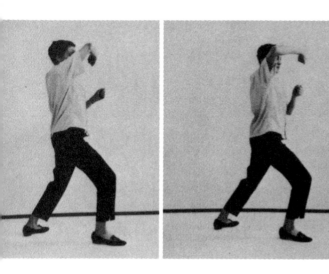

Form 48 (plate 4)   Form 48 (plate 5)

Lesson Fourteen:

49. Kick Upward with Right Foot. Weight shifts to left foot. Right foot steps back to left foot, right toe only touching floor. Legs bend, body lowers, as arms open outward and circle down around knees, palms open and facing in, right hand crossed over left. Body straightens and arms open at shoulder level and right foot kicks up, returning only toe to floor.

50. Strike Opponent's Ears with Both Fists. Right knee lifts and arms close in, in front of body, palms facing

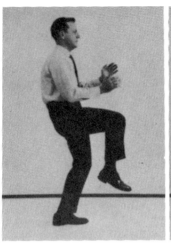 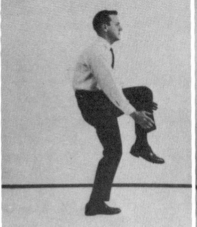 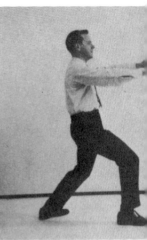

Form 50: *Strike Opponent's Ears with Both Fists*

Form 50 (plate 2)

Form 50 (plate 3)

each other. Arms descend on either side of right knee, palms still facing in. Right foot steps forward, weight shifting to right foot, right knee bending, as arms circle back, outward and forward, at head level, fists almost touching at arm's length in front of face, as though to strike the ears of an opponent. The fists are palm down.

NOTE:

When right foot steps forward, be sure to step heel first, since there is a tendency to let the foot return to the floor, toe first. When striking forward with both fists, be sure that the left leg is bent enough to keep the torso erect.

51. Turn Body and Kick Upward with Left Foot. Weight shifts to left foot. Body pulls back and arms open outward. Arms cross in front of chest, right hand outside, palms facing in, as body turns leftward to face east, turning on both heels at once, weight shifting to right foot as turn is completed. Arms open at shoulder level and left foot kicks up, returning only toe to floor.

NOTE:

This turn is made with feet apart. When the turn is completed, feet are in same relation to each other, but reversed, the left foot leading.

Form 51: *Turn Body and Kick Upward with Left Foot*

Form 51 (plate 2)

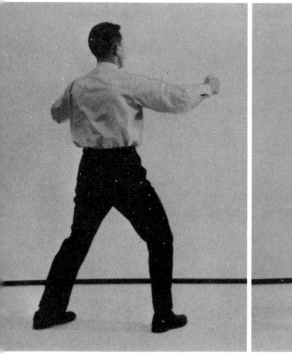
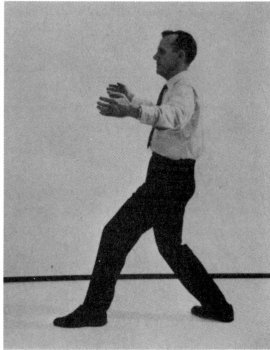

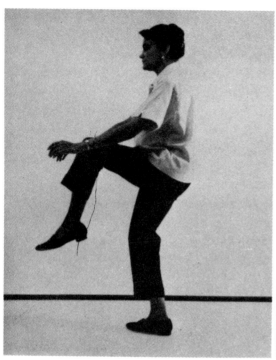
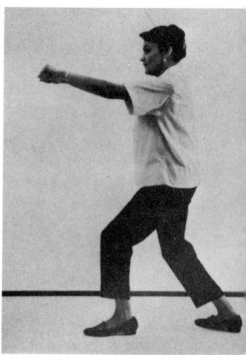

Form 52: *Strike Opponent's Ears*
with Both Fists

Form 52 (plate 2)

52. Strike Opponent's Ears with Both Fists. Left knee lifts and arms descend on either side of knee as in No. 50. Left foot steps forward (heel-first), and arms circle outward and forward as in No. 50.

✿   ✿   ✿

Lesson Fifteen:

53. Turn and Kick with Heel. Weight shifts to right foot. Left foot steps back to right foot, left toe only touching floor. Left arm comes in toward chest and body turns on sole of right foot, leftward to the west, arms closing during the turn, right over left. When turn is completed, arms open outward at shoulder level as left foot kicks out, heel leading as in No. 41.

54. Brush Knee and Twist Left. Hands form ball at right hip, left hand on top. Without returning to floor after kick, left foot steps southwest as left hand brushes past left knee and right hand circles back and pushes out over left knee as in No. 13. Direction is to the southwest.

NOTE:

At the beginning of this action, before stepping down with the left foot, the left leg bends at the knee, so that the step is a natural one, not a stiff one.

55. Strike Fist to Right. The same action as No. 18.

56. Step Forward and Punch. The same action as No. 19.

57. Cross Hands. The same action as No. 20. If Tai Chi is not to be continued into Section Three, Section Two ends here in the same way as Section One, indicated in No. 20.

Section Three

Lesson One:

🌿 **58. Carry Tiger to Mountain.** The same action as No. 21.

59. Push Up, Pull Back, Press Forward, Separate Hands and Push. The same action as No. 22.

60. Turn Body to Single Whip. The same action as No. 23. To the west.

61. Parting the Wild Horse's Mane Right. Body and both feet turn to right, left hand coming in toward chest, palm down, and right hand lowering to right side, palm forward, body swinging to right with swinging motion of arms. Right hand swings up before chest, palm down, and left hand lowers to left side, palm forward, body turning to left. Left hand swings up before chest, palm down, and right hand lowers to right side, palm forward, as body turns to right. Left foot takes small step back, weight shifting to left foot, and both hands pull down to form ball at left hip, right hand on top. Hands reverse, left hand coming to the top of the ball. Right foot steps northeast, weight shifting to right foot, right knee bending, as right hand rises over right knee, chin-high,

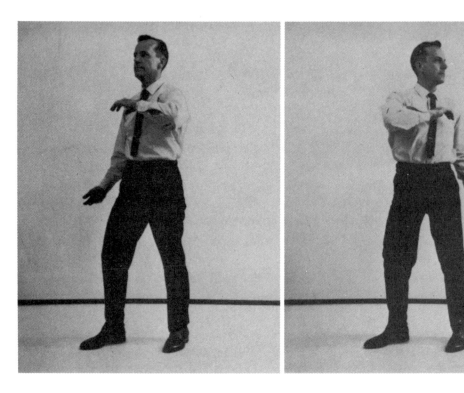

Form 61: *Parting the Wild Horse's Mane Right*

Form 61 (plate 2)

palm facing in, and left hand descends along left leg, palm facing back, as in Grasp Bird's Tail Right (No. 2).

NOTE:

In the beginning of this action, both feet turn together, left foot on heel and right foot on sole, until toes point slightly east of north, but not quite northeast. Feet are parallel and shoulder-width apart. Feet remain stationary in this position as body turns left and right. When body turns to right, weight shifts to right foot. When body turns to left, weight shifts

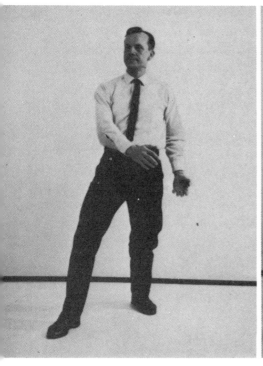

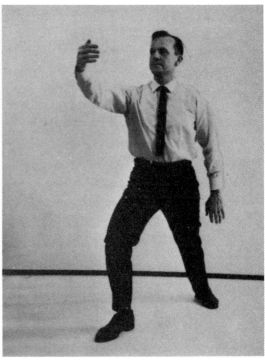

| Form 61 (plate 3) | Form 61 (plate 4) |

to left foot. The whole body turns with a swinging movement, arms swinging with body, as feet remain in place.

62. Parting the Wild Horse's Mane Left. Body and both feet turn to left (northwest), as right hand swings up before chest, palm down, and left hand turns palm forward at left side. Left hand swings up before chest, palm down, and right hand lowers to right side, palm forward, as body turns to the right. Right hand swings up before chest, palm down, as left hand lowers to left side, palm forward, body turning to the left. Right foot steps back, weight shifting to right foot, and hands pull down to form ball at right side, left hand on top. Hands reverse, right hand coming to top. Left foot steps northwest, weight shifting to left foot, left knee bending, as left hand rises over left knee, palm in, chin-high, and right hand descends along right leg, palm back, as in Grasp Bird's Tail Left (No. 3).

Form 62: *Parting the Wild*
Horse's Mane Left   **Form 62 (plate 2)**

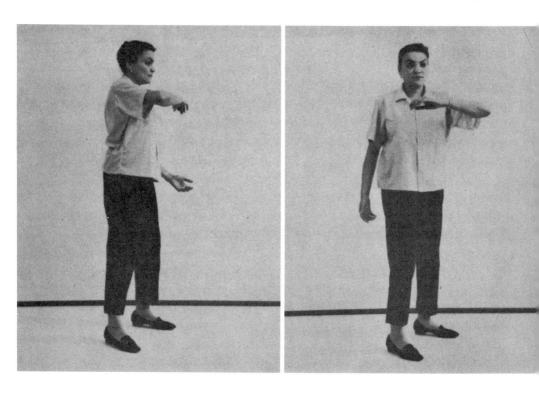

NOTE:

Although this is essentially the same action as No. 61, except that it faces a different direction, the arm movements are slightly different. When the hands pull down to the right side to hold the ball and then reverse, the left hand moves under the right elbow, palm up, before rising over left knee. The direction of the feet in this action is northwest.

Form 62 (plate 3)   **Form 62 (plate 4)**

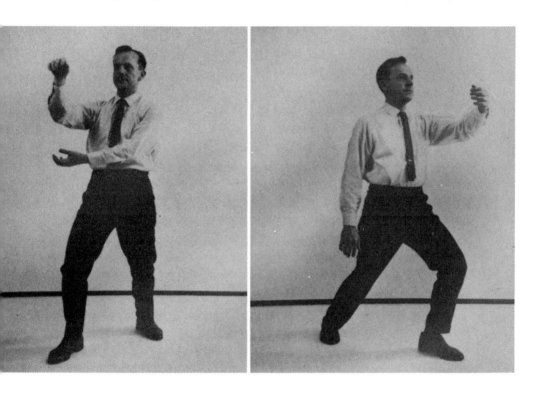

63. Parting the Wild Horse's Mane Right. Body and both feet turn to the right (northeast), as left hand swings in toward chest, palm down, and right hand, at right side, turns palm forward. Body turns to left as right hand swings up before chest, palm down, and left hand lowers to left side, palm forward. Body turns to right as left hand swings up before chest, palm down, and right hand lowers to right side, palm forward. Left foot takes small step back, weight shifting to left foot, and hands pull down to form ball at left side, right hand on top. Hands reverse. Right foot steps southeast, as right hand rises chin-high over right knee, palm in, and left hand descends along left leg, palm back.

✿   ✿   ✿

Lesson Two:

64. Grasp Bird's Tail Left. The same action as No. 3.

65. Push Up, Pull Back, Press Forward, Separate Hands and Push. The same actions as No. 4, No. 5, No. 6 and No. 7.

66. Turn Body to Single Whip. The same action as No. 8. To the southwest.

67. Fair Lady Works at Shuttles (1). Weight shifts to right foot. Left hand swings down under right elbow, palm up, as body turns northeast. Left foot turns on heel to northeast, then right foot turns on sole to northeast.

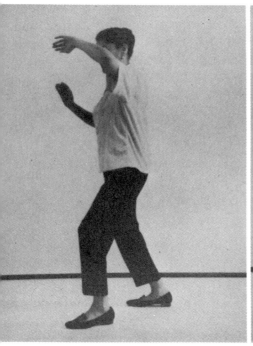 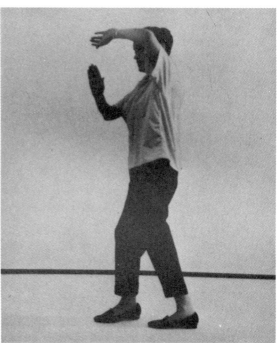

Form 67: *Fair Lady Works at Shuttles (1)*   Form 67 (plate 2)

Weight on right foot, left foot steps forward pointing east, weight shifting to left foot, left knee bending, as left arm rises to about one foot in front of forehead, palm facing in. Right foot steps up, crossing behind left foot, right toe pointing east, as left palm turns outward in front of forehead and right arm, elbow bent downward, pushes forward, palm slanting upward and outward, pointing under left arm to northeast, but not so far forward as left arm.

NOTE:

> This action is carefully synchronized, with left hand and left foot moving together and right hand and right foot moving together.

❀ ❀ ❀

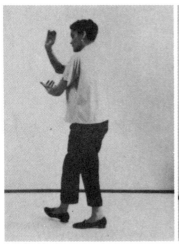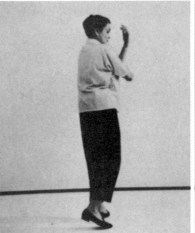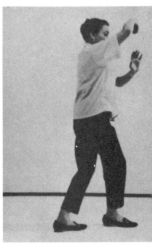

Form 68: *Fair Lady Works at Shuttles (2)*   **Form 68 (plate 2)**   **Form 68 (plate 3)**

Lesson Three:

68. Fair Lady Works at Shuttles (2). Weight shifts to right foot. Left hand swings down under right elbow, palm up, as left foot turns on heel to southwest. Right hand swings down under left elbow, palm up, as right foot turns and steps west, weight shifting to right foot, right knee bending. Right arm rises before forehead, palm curved and pointing down. Left foot steps up, crossing behind right foot, left foot also pointing west, as left hand pushes forward under right arm.

NOTE:

The right hand before the face is loosely fisted, pointing down, similar to the right hand position of Single Whip, except that fingers are not touching each other.

The palm does not turn outward as in No. 67. When the right foot is about to step, it must first swivel on ball of foot, in order to be in a position to step.

69. Fair Lady Works at Shuttles (3). Left hand swings under right elbow, palm up. Left foot steps forward and sideward, pointing west, weight shifting to left foot, left knee bending, and left arm rises before forehead, palm in. Left palm turns outward as right foot crosses behind left foot, right foot also pointing west, and right hand pushes forward under left arm.

Form 69: *Fair Lady Works at Shuttles (3)*

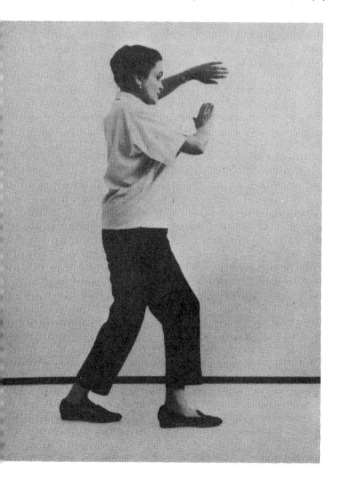

70. Fair Lady Works at Shuttles (4). Weight shifts to right foot. Left hand swings down under right elbow, palm up, as left foot turns on heel to northeast, weight shifting to left foot. Right hand swings under left elbow, palm up, as right foot turns and steps east, weight shifting to right foot, right knee bending as right arm rises before forehead, palm curved and pointing down. Left foot crosses behind right foot, pointing east, as left hand pushes forward under right arm.

* * *

Form 70: *Fair Lady Works*
at Shuttles (4)   **Form 70 (plate 2)**

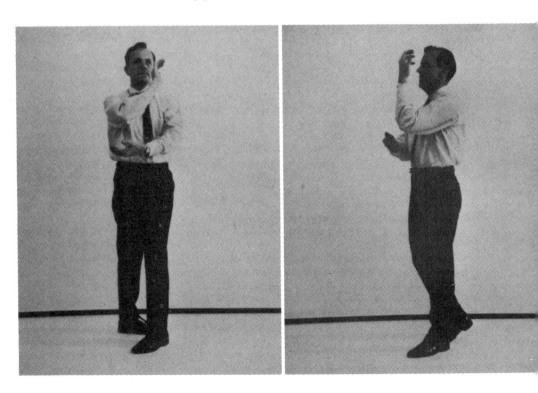

Lesson Four:

71. Grasp Bird's Tail Left. Left hand swings under right elbow, palm up. Left foot steps north, weight shifting to left foot, left knee bending, as left hand rises chin-high over left knee, palm in, and right hand descends along right leg, palm back.

Form 70 (plate 3)

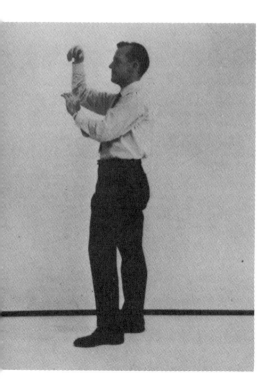

72. Push Up, Pull Back, Press Forward, Separate Hands and Push. The same action as No. 4, No. 5, No. 6 and No. 7.

73. Turn Body to Single Whip. The same action as No. 8. To the southwest.

74. Wave Hands Like Clouds. The same action as No. 36. It should be done four times here instead of six times, as in No. 36. Demonstrated here by a different student.

Form 74: *Wave Hands Like Clouds*

Form 74 (plate 2)

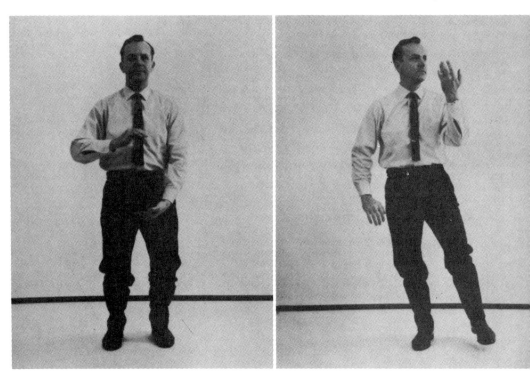

75. Single Whip. The same action as No. 37.

NOTE:

There is no new action in Lesson Four. However, the first three lessons of Section Three require considerable practice, and it is enough to add these movements to the sequence to be remembered, without learning a completely new action.

✿   ✿   ✿

Form 74 (plate 3)   **Form 74 (plate 4)**

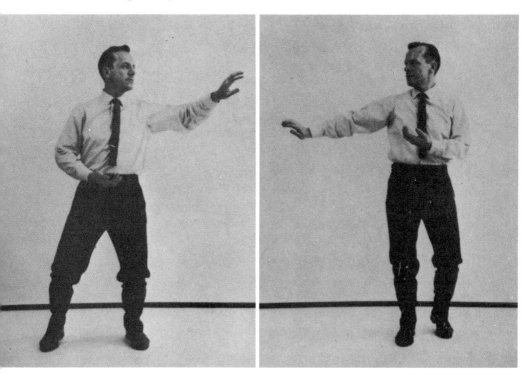

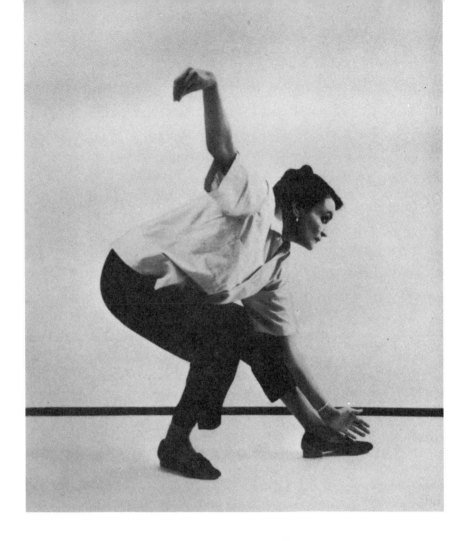

Form 76: Snake Creeps Down

Lesson Five:

76. Snake Creeps Down. Weight shifts to right foot. Right knee bends deeply, left leg straightening, as body lowers, sitting back on right leg. Body bends forward, weight still on right leg. Right arm remains stretched outward and upward in Single Whip position as left arm lowers and scoops down along inside of left leg, fingers pointing down, palm facing north.

NOTE:

In the beginning you will probably not be able to lower the body very much. Don't strain. The important thing is to maintain a comfortable balance, not to strive to get as low as possible.

✿   ✿   ✿

Lesson Six:

77. Golden Cock Stands on One Leg (1). Left knee bends. Weight shifts forward to left foot, as left arm scoops upward and body straightens. Right leg comes forward with knee lifted, and right arm comes forward, loose fist upward, palm facing left, elbow dropping to a point directly over raised right knee, left arm lowering to left side, palm back.

NOTE:

Right foot hangs loosely when right knee is lifted. In the beginning, if it is difficult to balance on the left leg while the right knee comes up, you can break the movement by resting the right toe lightly beside the left foot, before lifting the right knee.

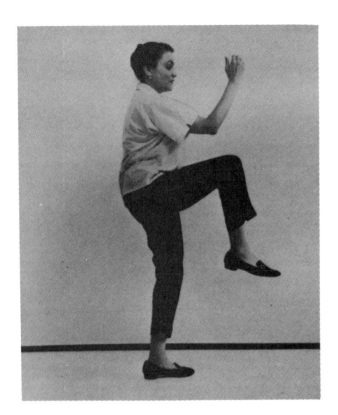

Form 77: Golden Cock
Stands on One Leg (1)

78. Golden Cock Stands on One Leg (2). Right foot steps backward and slightly to the right, weight shifting to right foot, right toe still pointing west. Left knee lifts and left arm comes up, loose fist upward, palm facing right, with left elbow directly over raised left knee, right fist lowering and loosening to open palm at right side, palm back.

NOTE:
> After right foot steps back, right arm and left arm move at the same time, fists passing each other as the left goes up and the right goes down.

❁　❁　❁

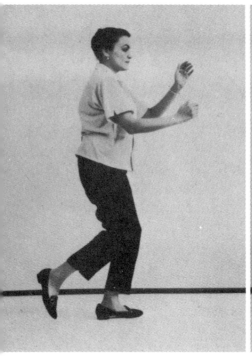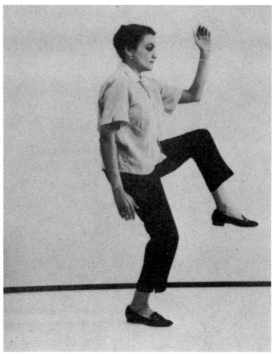

Form 78: Golden Cock
Stands on One Leg (2)

Form 78 (plate 2)

Lesson Seven:

79. Step Back and Repulse Monkey. Without returning to floor, left foot steps backward, left hand sinks beside left hip, palm up, as right hand circles back and pushes forward as in No. 25. Right foot steps back, then left foot steps back, with accompanying arm movements as in No. 25.

80. Slanting Flying. The same action as No. 26.

81. Raise Hands and Step Up. The same action as No. 27.

82. Stork Spreads Wings. The same action as No. 28.

✿   ✿   ✿

Lesson Eight:

83. Brush Knee and Twist Left. The same action as No. 11.

84. Needle at Sea Bottom. The same action as No. 30.

85. Raise Arms Like Fan. The same action as No. 31.

86. Turn and White Snake Puts Out Tongue. Hands move up, crossing above and before face, left hand over right, palms out. Arms make a descending circle to the sides, right hand forming loose fist. Meanwhile, body and feet turn to northeast, left foot turning on heel and right foot on sole. Hands come up in front of body, waist-high, left palm open and facing down, left hand a few inches above closed right fist which is turned palm upward. Right foot takes small step to southeast, weight shifting to right foot, right knee bending, as arms extend forward to east, right fist opening slowly to open palm facing up.

✿   ✿   ✿

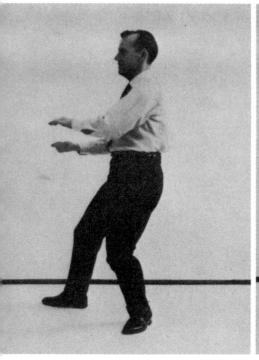
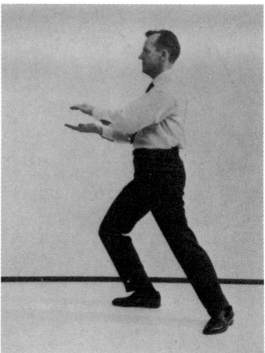

Form 86: *Turn and White Snake*
Puts Out Tongue

Form 86 (plate 2)

Lesson Nine:

87. Step Forward and Punch. The same action as No. 33, first shifting weight to left foot.

88. Push Up, Pull Back, Press Forward, Separate Hands and Push. The same action as No. 22.

89. Turn Body to Single Whip. The same action as No. 8. To southwest.

90. Wave Hands Like Clouds. The same action as No. 36. Four times.

✿   ✿   ✿

Lesson Ten:

91. Single Whip. The same action as No. 37.

92. High Pat on Horse. The same action as No. 38.

Form 93: *Separate Hands*

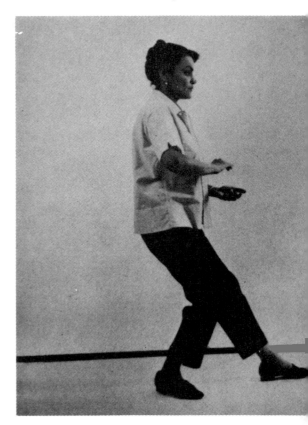

93. Separate Hands. Weight shifts to right foot and body pulls back as hands form ball close to abdomen, right hand on top. Body pushes forward, weight shifting to left foot, left knee bending, as hands, still holding ball, push forward to the west and then separate horizontally outward. As weight shifts back to right foot, body pulling back, hands close in front of chest, crossed at wrists, right over left, palms facing in. Left foot steps back to right foot, left toe only touching floor.

✿   ✿   ✿

Form 93 (plate 2)

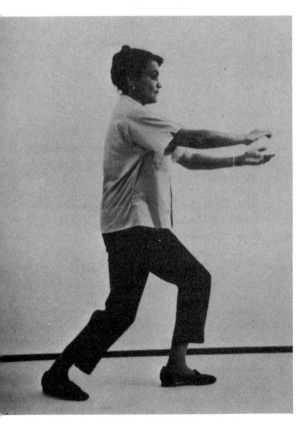

Lesson Eleven:

94. **Turn and Kick Sidewards.** This action is the same as No. 41 and No. 53, except that the kick with left foot is forward and then horizontally to the left before returning to the floor in the next action. Also the foot is in normal position, not with the heel leading as in No. 41 and No. 53.

95. (a) **Brush Knee and Twist Left and Right.** The same action as No. 42.
    (b) **Circle Hand and Punch in Middle.** The same action as No. 43, except that the punch is directed at a point just below waist level rather than downward toward foot.

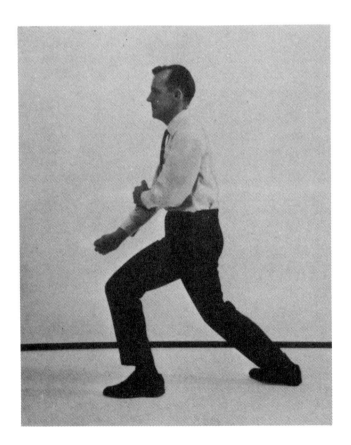

Form 95-b: *Circle Hand and Punch in Middle*

96. Push Up, Pull Back, Press Forward, Separate Hands and Push. The same action as No. 34.

✽ ✽ ✽

Lesson Twelve:

97. Turn Body to Single Whip. The same action as No. 8. To the southwest.

98. Snake Creeps Down. The same action as No. 76.

99. Step Up to Form Seven Stars. Body straightens up and hands form fists as weight shifts to left foot. Right foot steps forward, pointing west, weight shifting to right foot, as arms push forward crossed at wrists, left fist over right. Left fist faces in, right fist faces out.

✽ ✽ ✽

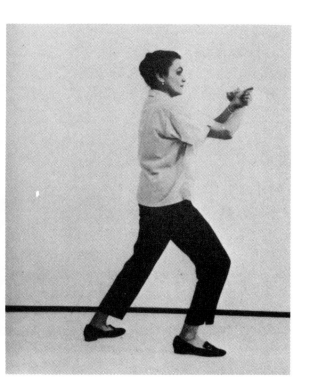

Form 99: *Step Up and Form Seven Stars*

Lesson Thirteen:

100. Kick Up with Right Foot. Weight shifts to left foot, body pulling back. Fists, still crossed, draw back close to body. Right foot kicks upward.

Form 100: *Kick Up with Right Foot*

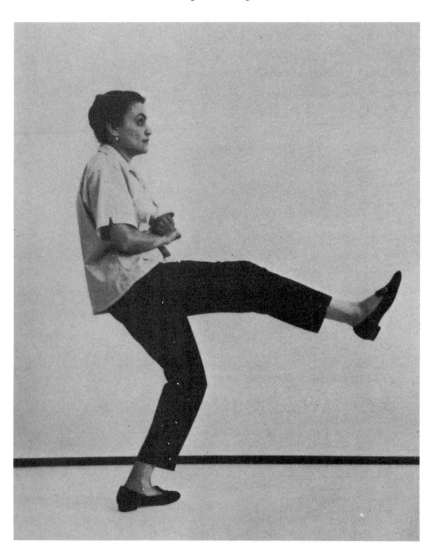

101. Retreat to Ride Tiger. Without returning to floor after kick, right foot steps backward a full step behind left foot, weight shifting to right foot. Fists open and right hand rises before forehead, palm down, fingers pointing left, and left hand drops to left side, palm back. Left foot lifts slightly, returning toe to floor. This position is similar to Stork Spreads Wings, No. 10.

✿   ✿   ✿

Form 101: *Retreat to Ride Tiger*

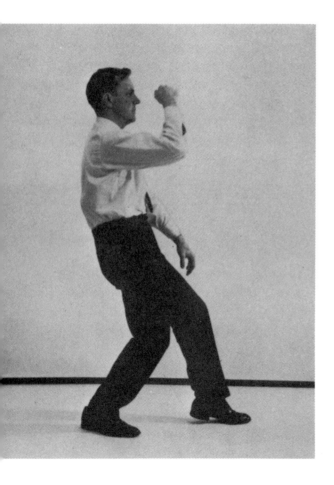

Lesson Fourteen:

102. Kick Up with Left Foot. Weight on right foot, left foot kicks upward, returning only toe to floor. Hands remain in same position as in No. 101.

103. Turn and Pat Foot. Right hand lowers to right side. Weight is on right foot. Left foot lifts from floor and left leg hangs straight, toe just barely off floor. Body turns to the right on the sole of right foot, turning completely around in three small turns, returning to face west again. Hands are hanging at sides during the turn. As turn is completed, hands stretch out chest-high in front of the body. Left foot steps down, parallel to right foot and weight shifts to left foot. Right foot kicks up between outstretched hands, and both hands touch right foot as it then moves sidewards toward right. Right foot returns to floor with only toe touching.

Form 103: Turn and Pat Foot   **Form 103 (plate 2)**   **Form 103 (plate 3)**

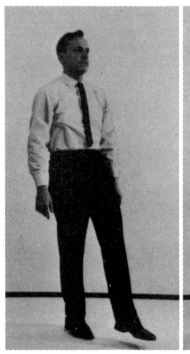
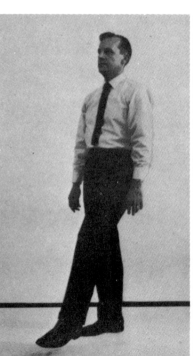
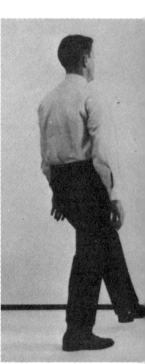

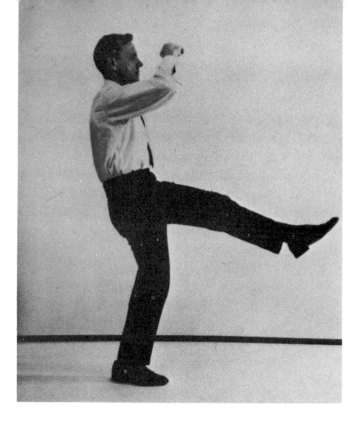

Form 102: *Kick Up*
with Left Foot

Form 103 (plate 4)

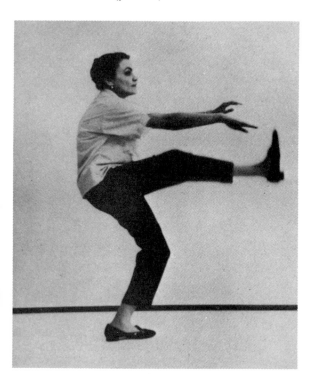

104. Shoot Tiger. Hands form fists. Weight on left foot, right foot steps northwest, weight shifting to right foot, right knee bending. Fists, held out at arm's length, move to the left, and then circle over in front of face to the right, right fist turning out in front of forehead and left fist, in punching position under right fist as in No. 48. Left fist is normal fist.

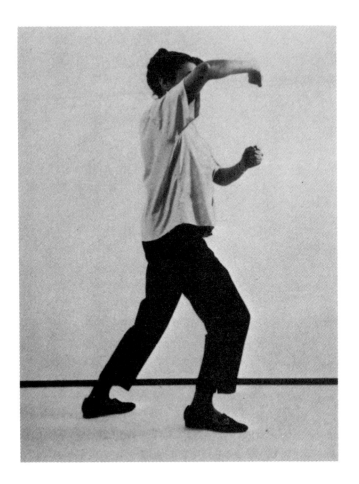

Form 104: *Shoot Tiger*

105. Strike Fist to Right. Left hand lowers to left side, palm back. Right fist circles down to abdomen, right arm continuing to circle clockwise to the left, up in front of face, and out to right (north). Head turns to north, eyes looking at fist.

106. Step Forward and Punch. Weight shifts to left foot and right foot takes small step to northwest, weight shifting to right foot, right knee bending, as right arm continues to circle down, fist coming up in front of body. Right arm, elbow bent, then draws back along right side, waist-high, as left arm swings up before chest, left palm facing in. Left foot steps southwest, weight shifting to left foot, left knee bending, as right arm curves up and forward straightening out at waist level, right fist punching to west, middle knuckle protruding. Left hand meets and rests on inside of right elbow.

107. Cross Hands. The same action as the first part of No. 20.

Form 107: *Cross Hands*   **Form 107 (plate 2)**

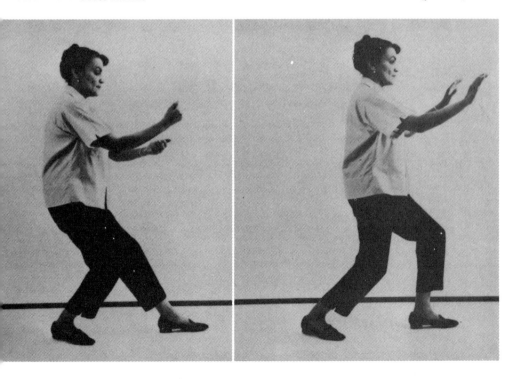

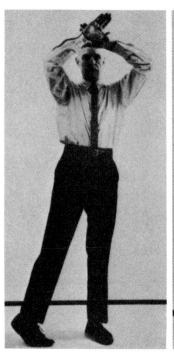 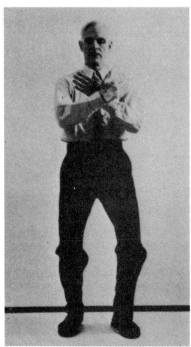 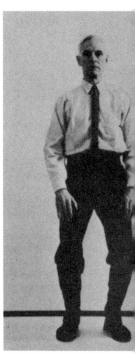

Form 108: End of
Tai Chi

Form 108 (plate 2)

Form 108 (plate

108. End of Tai Chi. Return to the opening position
as indicated in the last part of No. 20.

NOTE:
At the end you should find yourself in exactly the
same spot where you were when you started Tai Chi
in Form No. 1.

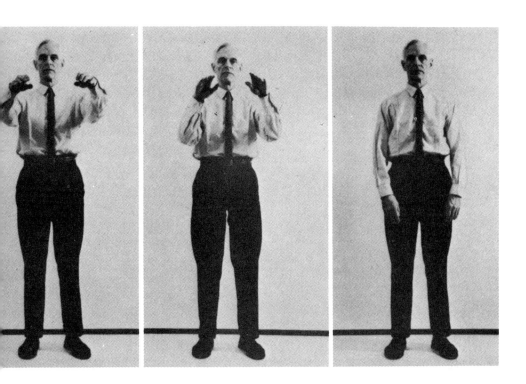

orm 108 (plate 4)   Form 108 (plate 5)   Form 108 (plate 6)

Short Tai Chi

It is essential to practice every day. Do not omit your daily practice of Tai Chi because of lack of time. If you do not have 14 or 15 minutes in the morning and evening, perform a shorter version. Do Section One and Section Two, or Section One and Section Three, or, if you have very little time, do just Section One, which takes about 4 minutes at a reasonably slow speed. Do not, however, do only Section Two or Section Three, as the slow, gentle beginning of Section One is necessary in the same way that a "warm-up" is necessary to athletes before undertaking more complicated activity.

Continuing with Tai Chi

The study of Tai Chi is a continuing experience. It is not over when you have memorized all the movements in the correct sequences. Further practice and study are most rewarding, as new concepts and illuminations emerge. When you feel comfortable in the practice of Tai Chi as described in these instructions, you may find it interesting and profitable to re-learn the entire series by reversing the direction.

Tai Chi to the Left

Instead of beginning the movements to the right with the first "Grasp Bird's Tail," turn and step to the left. All succeeding movements will then be to directions opposite to those indicated in these instructions, except those movements which face north or south. Even though the execution of the exercises in one direction only is considered to activate the muscles throughout the body, you may feel that certain muscles seem to be used more on one side of the body. In that case, practicing Tai Chi to the left as well as to the right would insure that both sides of the body receive the same amount of exercise.

Tai Chi with Speed

Additional variety can be obtained through varying the speed at which the series is practiced. Some medical authorities, as indicated in Part One of this book, favor the extreme slowness which develops sustained control of the muscles and is non-violent. They are even concerned about possible harmful effects of rapid exercise. Other authorities, as also indicated in Part One, recommend that the exercises be executed at a faster pace and emphasize the importance of rapid or vigorous exercise if it is built up to gradually enough. The speed at which you elect to perform should be governed by your own physical condition and state of health. The advice of your physician will be very useful.

If you practice in the morning just after arising, or at night just before retiring, it is recommended that at these times the series should be performed slowly, as mentioned earlier.

But at whatever speed you perform, you must keep in mind at all times that the speed should not change during the execution of the series. It must be even and uniform. The Chinese use the image of drawing silk from a cocoon. If you pull the silk out evenly, all the time at the same speed, it comes out easily, but if you pull slowly, then quickly, then slowly, the silk breaks.

To Advance with Tai Chi

Tai Chi is not a rigid, dogmatic, superimposed discipline. It adjusts and adapts to your own body. A tall man will not do it in exactly the same manner as a short man. A fat man will not look like a thin man. A man first recovering from a heart ailment will practice in a less vigorous fashion than an athlete who is accustomed to strenuous exercise. By practice, adjustment, and even experimentation, you will find the style most suitable for you. But in making personal adjustments, be very careful not to violate any of the basic principles of Tai Chi. For example, if you find that you have thoughtlessly fallen into the habit of practicing without keeping the knees bent, you would be advised to overcome this tendency and resume the practice with bending knees. The same holds true for the continuous shifting of weight from one foot to the other, and to the straight (but not rigid) back, the soft movements, etc. Refer often to the Ten Basic Rules on page 67. Even after you have learned the entire series and have been practicing it for months, it is well to read these pages again every few weeks, for there is a tendency to become sloppy if you do not constantly check yourself.

Handy Check-list of the 108 Forms

SECTION ONE

1. Beginning of Tai Chi.
2. Grasp Bird's Tail Right.
3. Grasp Bird's Tail Left.
4. Push Up.
5. Pull Back.
6. Press Forward.
7. Separate Hands and Push.
8. Turn Body to Single Whip.
9. Raise Hands and Step Up.
10. Stork Spreads Wings.
11. Brush Knee and Twist Left.
12. Play Guitar.
13. Brush Knee and Twist Left.
14. Brush Knee and Twist Right.
15. Brush Knee and Twist Left.
16. Play Guitar.

17. Brush Knee and Twist Left.
18. Strike Fist to Right.
19. Step Forward and Punch.
20. Cross Hands.

SECTION TWO

21. Carry Tiger to Mountain.
22. Push Up, Pull Back, Press Forward, Separate Hands and Push.
23. Turn Body to Single Whip.
24. Fist under Elbow.
25. Step Back and Repulse Monkey.
26. Slanting Flying.
27. Raise Hands and Step Up.
28. Stork Spreads Wings.
29. Brush Knee and Twist Left.
30. Needle at Sea Bottom.
31. Raise Arms Like Fan.
32. Turn Body and Strike Fist Back.
33. Step Forward and Punch.
34. Push Up, Pull Back, Press Forward, Separate Hands and Push.
35. Turn Body to Single Whip.
36. Wave Hands Like Clouds.
37. Single Whip.
38. High Pat on Horse.
39. Separate Right Foot.
40. Separate Left Foot.
41. Turn and Kick with Heel.
42. Brush Knee and Twist Left and Right.
43. Circle Hand and Punch Downward.
44. Turn Body and Strike Fist Back.
45. Step Forward and Punch.
46. Kick Upward with Right Foot.
47. Hit Tiger at Left.

SECTION TWO *(Cont.)*

48. Hit Tiger at Right.
49. Kick Upward with Right Foot.
50. Strike Opponent's Ears with Both Fists.
51. Turn Body and Kick Upward with Left Foot.
52. Strike Opponent's Ears with Both Fists.
53. Turn and Kick with Heel.
54. Brush Knee and Twist Left.
55. Strike Fist to Right.
56. Step Forward and Punch.
57. Cross Hands.

SECTION THREE

58. Carry Tiger to Mountain.
59. Push Up, Pull Back, Press Forward, Separate Hands and Push.
60. Turn Body to Single Whip.
61. Parting the Wild Horse's Mane Right.
62. Parting the Wild Horse's Mane Left.
63. Parting the Wild Horse's Mane Right.
64. Grasp Bird's Tail Left.
65. Push Up, Pull Back, Press Forward, Separate Hands and Push.
66. Turn Body to Single Whip.
67. Fair Lady Works at Shuttles (1).
68. Fair Lady Works at Shuttles (2).

69. Fair Lady Works at Shuttles (3).
70. Fair Lady Works at Shuttles (4).
71. Grasp Bird's Tail Left.
72. Push Up, Pull Back, Press Forward, Separate Hands and Push.
73. Turn Body to Single Whip.
74. Wave Hands Like Clouds.
75. Single Whip.
76. Snake Creeps Down.
77. Golden Cock Stands on One Leg (1).
78. Golden Cock Stands on One Leg (2).
79. Step Back and Repulse Monkey.
80. Slanting Flying.
81. Raise Hands and Step Up.
82. Stork Spreads Wings.
83. Brush Knee and Twist Left.
84. Needle at Sea Bottom.
85. Raise Arms Like Fan.
86. Turn and White Snake Puts Out Tongue.
87. Step Forward and Punch.
88. Push Up, Pull Back, Press Forward, Separate Hands and Push.
89. Turn Body to Single Whip.
90. Wave Hands Like Clouds.
91. Single Whip.
92. High Pat on Horse.
93. Separate Hands.
94. Turn and Kick Sidewards.
95. (a) Brush Knee and Twist Left and Right.
    (b) Circle Hand and Punch in Middle.

SECTION THREE *(Cont.)*

96. Push Up, Pull Back, Press Forward, Separate Hands and Push.
97. Turn Body to Single Whip.
98. Snake Creeps Down.
99. Step Up to Form Seven Stars.
100. Kick Up with Right Foot.
101. Retreat to Ride Tiger.
102. Kick Up with Left Foot.
103. Turn and Pat Foot.
104. Shoot Tiger.
105. Strike Fist to Right.
106. Step Forward and Punch.
107. Cross Hands.
108. End of Tai Chi.

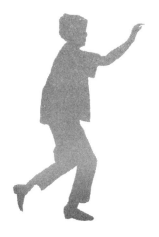

PART III

THE STORY
OF TAI CHI

How it can help
you Gain new benefits
from your practice

7

How it
all began

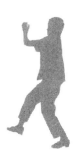

❧ Popular, if erroneous, theories concerning the origin of Tai Chi have often placed its beginnings in China a thousand years ago. An early Chinese way of life called Taoism had given birth to several historical movements which were by then well along in their development. The originators of Tai Chi are said to have been Taoist monks, who could quite logically be expected to have sought—even devised—some form of exercise as a relief from their long sedentary hours of meditation.

Male and Female

This is a nice notion, appealingly picturesque, and dovetailing in some ways with quantities of historical records of the Taoists and their customs. It is certain that they did, indeed, practice Tai Chi in one form or another. The concept of the Yin and the Yang, for example, a concept basic to Taoist thought, is demonstrated throughout the series of Tai Chi exercises.

Almost everyone is familiar with the symbol used by the Taoists to represent the synthesis of opposites, the circle divided into two equal parts by a serpentine line *(see illustration on opening page)*. The Yin (the dark half of the circle) represents the feminine and the negative. The Yang (the white half of the circle) represents the masculine and the positive. In many versions of the symbol there is a small white circle within the black area, and a small black circle within the white area. This indicates that everything includes its opposite. In every positive action there is some element of the negative and, conversely, no action is so negative that it completely leaves out the positive. The whole, therefore, contains an even balance of all opposites. The circle containing both halves represents the whole, continuing, unending, infinite.

The words "Tai Chi" in Chinese mean this whole circle made up of the Yin and the Yang. And the movements of Tai Chi supposedly follow these principles. Throughout the exercise opposites succeed each other in the progression of movement. Thus the hand which is above descends, and the hand which is down comes up. The leg which bears the weight (the strong, or Yang leg) becomes empty and weightless as the weight shifts to the other leg. The arms continually describe circles, large or small. The hands continually move through globe-holding positions—in theory, the hands are holding the Yin-Yang circle. No movement is complete in itself: it is always becoming something else, moving toward its opposite. And the end of every movement or gesture is not an end but the beginning of another movement.

Even a modest amount of research, however, quickly upsets the idea that it was the Taoists themselves who created Tai Chi as it is known and practiced today. It is also clear that the system had its origins much earlier than a thousand years ago.

The search for the real innovator leads one back over a trail that is at once fascinating, and exasperating. Authoritative early works on the subject are discouragingly scarce. Much of what was set down bears the clear stamp of fiction, and even in material which purports to be factual, repeated discrepancies cast doubt upon the care with which it was written.

Breathing and Butting

Certain early clues in authentic history, however, are of particular interest to the student today. There was, for example, a form of Taoist breathing exercise whose origin is unknown though it is mentioned in the official history of China which covers the period from earliest times up to 122 B.C. In conjunction with other forms of exercise, it was widely practiced. The importance of breathing as an integral part of Tai Chi we have already considered. (*See pages 15, 18-24, 67, 68-69.*)

Another type of gymnastics had earlier been inaugurated by a legendary emperor belonging to some ancient dynasty, as a method of improving the health of his people after a great flood. It was he who first compared an unexercised body to stagnant water.

In the era between 722 B.C. and 484 B.C., a kind of exercise which was also a sport came into being. It was called "butting" and consisted of just what the word implies.

Imitation of
Animal Movements

Much later than the first beginnings we have been looking at, a famous surgeon, who was born in 190 A.D., became the exponent of a systematic exercise. His biography appearing in the official history of the era between 25 B.C. and 265 A.D. contains this statement by him:

> The ancients practiced the bear's neck, the fowl's twist, swaying the body, and moving the joints to prevent old age and achieve longevity. I have a system of exercises . . . which are the tiger, the deer, the bear, the monkey and the bird. It removes disease, strengthens the legs, and ensures good health.

The reference to the "ancients" may have included the originators of a famous system known as the Five Animal Frolics. These came into being during the time which we would call the beginning of the Christian era. Like the earlier Taoist exercise, the Five Frolics combined breathing movements with their animal movements.

Tai Chi also, it should be remembered, according to long tradition, derives in part from the imitation of animal movements. This accounts for the extraordinary range of muscle-group combinations which are brought into play, as opposed to what happens in the ordinary calisthenics with which we are familiar. These by comparison proceed according to limited diagrams of the body's capabilities.

There is another especially important aspect of this early inspiration from animals. Tai Chi, as we have seen, must be done in an easy, relaxed way throughout. To relax, however, does not mean you should become a bag of bones. Real relaxation involves absorption in what you are doing. Observe a cat or dog at rest as the Chinese fathers of this exercise must shrewdly have observed many an animal, and you will see what true relaxation is; the dog and cat are completely relaxed, yet they are still capable of making sudden definite movements.

And also keep in mind that relaxation is not accomplished by straining for it. The dog or cat does not labor at it. It is a little like trying desperately to go to sleep; you usually find that trying only makes it more difficult. Do not worry if you feel you are not sufficiently relaxed right away. You will be when, in the easeful manner of animals, you become involved in what you are doing, you are at one with it.

The practice of the eminent surgeon's system based on the tiger, the deer, the bear, the monkey and the bird is not common today. The practice of two other therapeutic exercises, however, does currently exist. First is the doctrine of relaxing tension, which is usually attributed to Bodhidharma, the founder of Zen Buddhism. The other is the eight-fold movement pattern, whose origin is often disputed.

Our 108 Forms and the 37 Actions

One other figure of early history should be mentioned here because he has a special interest for present-day students of Tai Chi. We read a most astonishing bit about him in a twelfth-century compilation of biographies which covers the era 618 A.D. to 690 A.D. during which he lived. It says there that he:

> . . . abstained from cereals in order to attain immortality and often went without food. He was seven feet six inches in height.

His beard was so long that it reached his navel, while his hair touched his feet. He traveled as fast as a horse.

The descriptions in this old book are not mere exaggerations but figures of speech and a representative style of classical Chinese. For if we should interpret literally the comment that he was seven feet six inches tall—with the calculation that one Chinese foot equalled 14.1 English inches—then the man we are talking about would be 8.96 feet, which even as a "tall story" would have to be taken with more than a grain of salt, or sticking to the point, with more than a cubit or two of credulity!

To this long-beard, whatever his height, is usually attributed an exercise system made up of 37 movements or forms. The fact that he kept to a peculiar diet which was followed by a certain wing of the Taoists may lead one to believe that he also practiced their form of breathing exercise mentioned earlier. In any case this Taoist exercise came later to be called by the same name as his system and was likewise comprised of 37 movements.

As I have pointed out in Part One of this book, if we examine closely the movements of Tai Chi—which consist of 108 forms to be executed by turn in an unbroken flowing series—and delete the repeated motions and the similar ones, there is a remainder of 37 basic movements. It is possible therefore that the bearded dieter may be credited with the transmission of an ancient exercise down to the present.

Many other persons are mentioned by modern writers as having been either transmitters or inventors of Tai Chi, but the real existence of such people or their claim to any place in history is more than doubtful.

This brings us in the next chapter, then, to the man whose name predominates among all others brought to light thus far as the true originator of Tai Chi.

8

The search for the mysterious old man

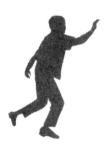

The words "Tai Chi," we have seen, in Chinese mean the symbol of the whole circle with its two necessary and complementary parts: the masculine and the feminine, or the positive and the negative, the Yin and the Yang. But the full name of the system of exercise we are practicing happens to be "Tai Chi Chuan."

"Chuan" becomes an important word in our search when we try to follow the mysterious path which leads to the discovery of the founding father of this calisthenic. Literally "chuan" in Chinese means "fist." If from this we proceed to conjure up in our own terms some notion of "fisticuffs" or "pugilism," mixed in with images of Jack Dempsey, Harry Greb or Sonny Liston, we shall be far off the track. The Chinese idea of "chuan" as combat involves, rather, the use of the entire physical self, absolutely every part of it, nothing excluded.

Tai Chi and Self-Defense

Pugilism, in this sense of exercise for the total physical being, in China became combined with certain principles of how to harmonize antagonistic movements both within oneself and in relation to an opponent. And such principles were gained or refined through application of the Tai Chi circle and what it stood for as the balance of opposing forces. Sometimes the "chuan" or combat was meant as between human opponents; sometimes the opponent was spiritual. It can refer to the physical self in its handling of any objective situation. Either way, this aspect of Tai Chi played a significant role in the development of the exercise as it has come down to us.

Chang San-feng, Tai Chi's Originator

Let us keep it in mind as we look briefly at some of the clues pointing to the identity of the elusive architect of Tai Chi. The evidence, far-flung in geography and widely scattered through time, all seems to point conclusively to one man. His name is Chang San-feng. There are, indeed, many scholars who have been content simply to credit him as the originator without considering any of the figures who may have come before or after.

In the official combination atlas-chronicle of one province in China, there appears the biography of a certain local dignitary who was "skilled in boxing." The name of his instructor in the pugilistic art is given. "According to him," the venerable record continues, "this art of boxing was originated [during the era between 910 A.D. and 1279 A.D.] by Chang San-feng," whom it identifies as an alchemist residing in the mountains.

In one old compilation of essays, the author includes an epitaph that refers to the "esoteric style" of boxing. This style, we are told, "which was started [during the same era mentioned above] by Chang San-feng, utilizes the principles of activating motion from calm or stillness. It teaches that when attacked, one should be prepared to place oneself out of reach."

Still another source, a collection of biographical notes about chivalrous persons, belongs to what the Chinese call "wild history," a type of record which for all its color and interest is not regarded as trustworthy. It reports: "The reputation of Chang San-feng of [the same era given again] who advocated the esoteric style of boxing, is spread throughout the empire."

One twentieth-century expert, in presenting a number of his own questionable "facts," has even elaborated upon Chang San-feng's father. "He was strong, trustworthy, and quite a remarkable person," we are told. When a three-category program was devised for "gathering together talented men," he "went for the examination and was immediately selected. It was a pity that he was indifferent and did not want to serve the government; thus he retired to the countryside where he died."

A fascinating portrait of the recluse himself emerges

from a few important sources. The official history of the era which runs from 1368 A.D. to 1644 A.D. claims him as its own and goes on:

> He was tall and had an imposing appearance. He bore the classical signs of longevity which were the elements of the tortoise and the crane. He had large ears and round eyes. His beard bristled with fury, like the blade of a halberd. In the winter or in summer he wore only a single garment and a matted hat. He either ate a great deal or else he would go for days without food. He could travel very rapidly, and go many miles in a single day. He was very virtuous and often laughed and giggled, so that no one who was near him could remain melancholic. He often visited the . . . mountains with his disciples. There he built a grass hut and took residence.

In 1391 A.D., the chronicle continues, the Emperor "heard of his name and ordered messengers who fruitlessly searched for him."

The Secret of Immortality

A convincing firsthand description is also offered by a contemporary scholar of this era, who refers to him as "the immortal Chang." Observing the father of Tai Chi as he was being led by a servant, the man writes, "I saw him then. His beard, whiskers, and the hair on his temples were full and bristling. He curled his hair in a ball on top of his head." The same witness tells us, "The Emperor granted him a title of honor, conferring upon him the title 'the wise and illustrious spiritual man who understands the occult.'"

From all the scattered scraps of information available about him two main conclusions concerning Chang San-feng may be reached. First, the historical period during which he lived may perhaps be narrowed down to the one which extends between the years 1260 A.D. and 1368 A.D. Secondly, he was in all likelihood a Taoist whose development of Tai Chi was bound up with the search for the elixir of life, or the secret of immortality. He was called "the immortal Chang," and the Emperor conferred upon him the title of a spiritual man who has attained the

Way, or Tao, and henceforth is moved only by an impulse operating through him.

Effortlessness—
the Key to Tai Chi

From this latter characteristic of the illustrious man who invented Tai Chi, the student today may derive a modest though highly useful lesson. For it is a practical and not-at-all occult matter that an easeful and relaxed quality of *effortlessness* becomes more and more the experience of anyone who practices the exercise over a period of time. You do not try and strain, strain and try. You do not drive yourself at all.

It will be helpful to remember this during your practice. Avoid thinking that you must make your body perform certain actions. Rather let these actions happen, as it were, through the medium of your body. To borrow a manner of expression that Chang San-feng would have approved, it is not you "doing" it. What it seems and feels like is that "it" is doing it through you. The same thing, as pointed out in an earlier chapter, should be true of your breathing which is not forced in any way but occurs naturally in accompaniment with the actions.

As far as possible I have phrased all the instructions in Part Two to try to indicate this sense that the actions accomplish themselves. "Arms raise slowly" is the way the wording usually runs, for example, instead of "Raise your arms slowly." You may also be assisted in this basic ease and effortlessness by the postural image of Tai Chi (*see pages 60-62*)—thinking of yourself as a marionette which dangles from, and whose movements are smoothly operated by, strings outside its control.

9

A 400-year
secret

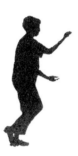

❧ In this book we are learning to do the classic Tai Chi which is sometimes more precisely designated as the Yang School. How did this ancient tradition come to acquire this additional name? It is so remembered today in honor of an amazing man who skillfully rescued the old exercise and restored it to public knowledge after it had been locked away, a carefully kept secret, from the world for more than 400 years.

This strange state of affairs came about not long after the death of Tai Chi's founding father, Chang San-feng. Tradition relates that the art was passed on to his foremost student who is supposed to have lived during the same period. There is actually no definite proof that this student lived at all but two basic writings on Tai Chi are attributed to him. (These are given, II and III in the Appendix, *pages 206-212.*)

The Northern School and the Southern School

After the death of this legendary disciple, two of his own devoted followers began to quarrel about the interpretation of the doctrines. This momentarily brought about a kind of civil war in the Tai Chi movement, resulting in a Northern School and a Southern School. The Confederate school, however, lasted for a very brief span, in the epochal terms by which such things are measured in Chinese history. And it was from the victorious Union forces that the exercise was passed on to a family clan by the name of Chen, who lived in a province called Honan. The members of this family monopolized and kept Tai Chi a secret for fourteen generations.

How the Chens Kept "The Secret"

How was such a thing possible? Mainly it was because of the stringent laws which the Chens laid down in order to conceal this treasure from the rest of the world. These rules forbade the teaching of Tai Chi to anyone outside the clan. No one was allowed to perform the exercises in public, nor to engage in any occupation which necessitated the use of its skills. It was also forbidden to teach anyone within the clan whose character was considered doubtful.

After 420-odd years of this unique monopoly there appeared a definite split within the Chen family as to the ideology governing Tai Chi. One faction which reacted somewhat against the age-old principles was termed the "new method." The other which insisted on the orthodox interpretation was termed the "old method." The member of the Chen family who held the fort both as fosterer and instructor of the "old method" was a man known for determination and strong principle, and for a nature which was very stern and upright. (His father and two uncles skilled in the arts of Tai Chi were often referred to as the "three heroes.") Fittingly, people nicknamed him "Strait-jacket Chen."

Owing to the conservative structure of Chinese society and the insistent hold of the way in which the Chen clan had always practiced, the precepts of the "new method" were much frowned upon. On the other hand, the system of the orthodox school was widely followed among the Chens. And it was from none other than the prestigious founder and chief exponent of the "old method," Strait-jacket Chen himself, that a daring young outsider managed to wrest the long-kept secret and give it to the world. Of all the old patriarch's many pupils, it turned out, the most notable was to be a man who formed no part of the family circle. His name was Yang Lu-chan.

How "The Secret" Was Revealed to the World

According to the records, this late-appearing Prometheus in Tai Chi history was born at the close of the eighteenth century and spent most of his youth in the country, his ancestors having traditionally been farmers. Small and slender, he nonetheless took an active interest in strenuous activities, and in the art of self-defense. His father engaged a master boxer to instruct him. The man taught the youth various types of exercises, including a system of self-defense which the student quickly mastered.

He also told him of an art called Tai Chi Chuan, but mentioned that it was impossible for an outsider to learn it. Yang pressed for more information, and his teacher told him that it was a closely guarded secret of the Chen clan in Honan province, and that the foremost master, at the time, was old Strait-jacket Chen. Yang Lu-chan was intrigued, and departed for Honan to investigate for himself.

On his arrival in the province he was told in what place the Chen household was located. He went there at once, pretended to be a household servant in search of work, and was immediately hired. Soon he had the run of the house, and discovered where the clansmen were practicing Tai Chi. Secretly he spied on them, and began practicing on his own.

One night, while going through the exercises, he was discovered by the master, old Strait-jacket Chen himself, who although seemingly provoked at what he saw, was impressed by Yang Lu-chan's skillful execution of the movements. He decided to make a radical departure from tradition and accept the youth as a pupil.

With this careful instruction from the master, Yang Lu-chan mastered the techniques of Tai Chi Chuan. And the master was so overwhelmed that he kept nothing from the young student. Yang Lu-chan continued his study for many years. At this time his mentor, devoted to the orthodox interpretation of the ancient art, told Yang Lu-chan that the Tai Chi Chuan that he had learned had deviated far from its original concept. He pointed out that Tai Chi had originally been an exercise for therapeutic benefits, and that it was slowly deteriorating into a sport and a form of self-defense. Yang Lu-chan thereupon began to study the basic concepts and philosophy of Tai Chi. Like his master, he went back to the original concepts expressed by Chang San-feng and also in the two treatises supposed to have been written by the foremost pupil of the old originator. Because of his remarkable achievement, Strait-jacket urged him to go to the capital, which was then Peking, to propagate the art.

The First School

In Peking, Yang Lu-chan promptly set up a school and gave instruction, but only to those whose character he approved. There are many stories of his struggles in Peking while trying to establish a school. One such story recorded in a chronicle of Tai Chi relates that:

> While Yang Lu-chan was residing in Peking there was a famous master-boxer who, after hearing that there was a person in Peking who was trying to inaugurate a new school of self-defense, proceeded to seek him out and ask for a bout. When he first approached Yang Lu-chan, he was very courteously received, and upon asking for a bout . . . was given a prompt refusal. The master boxer thought that Yang Lu-chan was afraid of him and repeatedly pressed the issue. Realizing that there was no other alternative, Yang Lu-chan reluctantly accepted the challenge. When the master boxer inquired about the conditions of fighting, Yang Lu-chan, smiling, said, "Why don't you just punch me three times?" When the master boxer heard him, he was overjoyed. Immediately he proceeded to deliver a severe blow at him. However, as the punch was being delivered, Yang Lu-chan gave an inadvertent laugh which put the master boxer off his feet.

Another story tells us:

> On another occasion while Yang Lu-chan was strolling near the riverside, there were two master boxers who, having heard of his fame, decided to attack him from the rear. With his back turned towards them, the two master boxers rushed upon him, whereupon Yang Lu-chan, sensing an attack, inclined his body slightly and sent the two master boxers sailing into the river.

There were, no doubt, many challenges with boxers in the Peking area, and Yang Lu-chan was popularly called "Yang the Unsurpassed."

By combining the early concepts of a therapeutic exercise and the later concepts of self-defense, Yang Lu-chan, although not deviating from the traditional concepts handed down to him by his instructor, thus started a school which—though quite classic—was named after him, the Yang School.

Carrying on the Ancient Tradition

After his death in 1872 at the age of 74, the Great Restorer left two sons, carefully instructed by their father to carry on the ancient tradition which he had single-handed retrieved from the confines where a single clan, huddling protectively over it for 400 years, had kept it fast imprisoned. Further restoring and wisely preserving it, Yang is remembered as the dauntless seeker who bequeathed Tai Chi to the larger outside world.

10

On to
America!

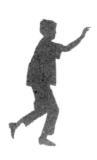

❧ From the two sons of the Great Restorer may be traced the whole, vast, proliferating development of classic Tai Chi in the modern world right up to the present. In the order in which they had been born they were often referred to by contemporaries as "Mr. Number Two" and "Mr. Number Three." (A first son, "Mr. Number One," had died in early youth.) The younger of them lived till 1917, the year of America's entry into World War I. His death then, at the age of 75, was proclaimed a great loss to teaching since "Mr. Number Three" is said to have equalled his father, the redoubtable Yang himself, in the execution of Tai Chi.

Tai Chi in Modern Times

Whoever glances at the subsequent history of the exercise from that time on down to its prevalence in the Chinese world today is confronted with a ludicrously complicated spectacle of genealogy. First of all, descending from the original two sons in ever-widening rivulets is the blood succession of their own sons, and the sons of those sons, and then *their* sons, and so on. Next there are the pupils (some of them prize pupils) of the original two sons, and the pupils of those pupils, and then the pupils of *their* pupils, and so on. Frequently the two modes of lineage intermix. We have sons of pupils of sons, and pupils of sons of pupils.

The Western observer of Tai Chi among the modern Chinese had better curb his smile. It is not entirely a matter of Chinese custom. For it was not too long ago that among ourselves there was a similar vogue among music students for establishing their skill by this kind of convoluted pedigree. A keyboard friend might tell you with the utmost gravity that his own teacher was a student of a teacher who was Leschetizky's prize pupil. Or a screeching woman acquaintance might boast that she was studying with a teacher who had been the student of the teacher who coached Nellie Melba.

Amusing and even impressive as such references may be, this kind of thing provides sparse pickings as the stuff of history. It will be enough for most of us simply to know that the ancient exercise culminated in a kind of prolific Malthusian progression after it had once been found again by Yang.

Widespread Adoption of Tai Chi

The advent of cheap commercial printing also contributed to this great expansion in its practice. Manuals of instruction in Tai Chi thus became readily available in remote regions which happened to have no sons of pupils of pupils in their vicinity from whom to learn. A final touch in the spread of the exercise was its widespread adoption into many school systems as the required or optional form of physical training. This occurred at almost every level of education from childhood to college.

Today, as mentioned in earlier chapters, it is practiced everywhere both on Taiwan and the Chinese mainland. An official manual of instruction in the classic Yang teaching has been issued by the Division of Tai Chi Chuan of the Department of Physical Education for the Peoples' Government of Communist China. Since 1953 the All-China Athletic Federation has been actively encouraging the practice of Tai Chi among its various organizations. Teachers have also been invited by North Vietnam to visit and give lessons there. The Soviet specialist on sports physiology, I. Baichenko, who before the Sino-Soviet break was advisor to the Peking Physical Culture Institute, conceived a very high respect for the health-giving and therapeutic value of the traditional exercise.

Other Forms of Tai Chi

Besides the classic Yang widely practiced everywhere, there are three minor-league forms of Chinese exercise more sparsely in evidence at the present time and also called Tai Chi. Of these little need be said here—with one exception. A special note of warning about this one is in order for the benefit of Americans.

The instructions given in this book, as well as all the medical and scientific appraisals cited, apply specifically and only to the classic Tai Chi, which is designated more precisely as the Yang tradition. What is said throughout is not meant to, and does not, apply to all the other extant forms of Chinese calisthenics which are also often simply called "Tai Chi" without differentiation. One of these in particular, a quite recent offshoot of the classic exercise, and known as Wu, after the man who thought it up, is occasionally seen in this country. It is entirely different in movement and has certain disadvantages from the viewpoint of health benefit.

A technical evaluation of this system and its shortcomings would be out of place in the present book. But how it came into being forms a peripheral incident in the history of Tai Chi and may be included briefly here. Its inventor was the student of a teacher who was a student of "Mr. Number Two." Dissatisfied with the instruction which he had received, he made radical changes in the execution of all the movements, emerging with a totally different system of exercises all his own, and started a new school named after himself, called the Wu school.

Commenting upon this recent development, Dr. William C. Hu, Tai Chi scholar and Librarian at the Asia Library of the University of Michigan, remarks:

> After a continuous tradition of several centuries, it seems unfortunate that a break should again occur in the concepts of Tai Chi. It can now be considered a radical break—a serious departure—since the changes inaugurated by Wu in the movements of the art were without any strongly necessitated principles other than personal style.

It is most important for the student of Tai Chi, then, always to be alert and certain that he is dealing with the classic, or Yang, form of the exercise. Since that is the form generally being taught throughout the country today, nine chances out of ten it will be Yang that he will encounter, whether in joining a social practice group, or in forming one of his own, or in seeking a teacher with whom to carry on some advanced study. But he should, none the less, take every care at the beginning. Otherwise he may find himself winding up in needless disappointment and failure through lack of caution at the outset in investigating just what it is that he is about to learn.

The so-called Wu stylization—though sometimes confusingly presented as the "ancient" form—is, rather, a highly artificial and less effective patchwork, professedly inspired by it. And in the Western terms of physical and mental self-improvement which concern us, Mr. Wu's tricksy modern brainchild is scarcely to be compared in value with the old, long-time empirically tested system of movement which is embodied in the true, earlier Tai Chi.

The Tai Chi Boom
in America

The present Tai Chi boom in America as reported in everything from local newspapers to national TV and certain popular journals is often attributed to me because of my teaching, writing, and lecturing. But the initial transplantation of Tai Chi to America may be traced mainly to other persons, some of whom first instructed large numbers of American students in the exercise and one who taught widely among the various Chinese groups throughout the country. All had wide followings, and are together responsible for first setting in motion the Tai Chi study movement here.

As early as 1935 there is a Pathé newsreel which shows a West Coast teacher leading a group of students in practice outdoors. In 1948 a well-known experimental cinematographer, the late Maya Deren, made a film of which one section, in a sequence of rather freewheeling and fantastic improvisations by Chao-li Chi, took off from

Tai Chi. The film, first exhibited at New York's Province-town Playhouse that same year, was afterwards shown at universities and in various little theaters throughout the country. And as it became known, lectures about and demonstrations of the original calisthenic itself were held under several auspices. Private lessons were taken by a considerable number of people. It was not till 1961, with the new renaissance of interest in the exercise, that the Tai Chi Institute of America was founded in New York by Betty Cage and myself (on a nonprofit basis).

Not much is known concerning the real Tai Chi pioneer in America, who trained the greater part of the Chinese now teaching in local communities throughout this country. Born in 1885 this man, named Choy Hak Pang, came to the United States in 1941 or 1942 and remained here for a period of about seven years. Here he taught many students in San Francisco, Los Angeles and also in New York. Returning to Hong Kong in 1948, where he lived till his death, he became widely known as a teacher, and his book on Tai Chi published in 1956 had wide circulation there. Of the thousand students he is reported to have taught, a large number were scattered through this country. Choy Hak Pang died in 1958.

By his Chinese students in America, he is remembered with great warmth. Commonly upon visiting their homes or clubhouses, one sees upon the wall a picture taken during his American sojourn. Usually in such pictures the familiar smiling face of the Tai Chi instructor is shown surrounded by the equally smiling faces of a class of devoted students.

Though he taught no Americans himself, he carried on an extensive training program among the Chinese in this country, many of whom later became teachers. Because he nurtured the seed that spread, it is Choy Hok Pang who must be remembered as the father of Tai Chi in America.

After Choy Hak Pang, Tai Chi has been put under the microscope for the kind of scholarly study expected in this country. The health writer Jane Brody offers two intriguing examples.

In a fifteen-week study sponsored by the National Institute on Aging and published in the *Journal of the American Geriatrics Society* in May 1996, Dr. Steven L. Wolf, a rehabilitation medicine specialist at Emory University School of Medicine, randomly assigned 215 people 70 and older to three groups. One group, says Brody, "took weekly Tai Chi Lessons and practiced on their own twice daily. Another met to discuss issues important to the elderly and were told to continue their usual exercise. The third got balance-training."

The results? Blood pressure fell among those doing Tai Chi. Their grip strength increased, and the participants' sense of control over their lives improved. "But most important," notes Brody, "when followed for up to 17 months after the training period ended, the members of the Tai Chi group had reduced their risk of falls nearly in half."

The other study Brody cites was done by researchers at the University of Connecticut and showed that leg strength increased in people over 75 who were trained in Tai Chi.

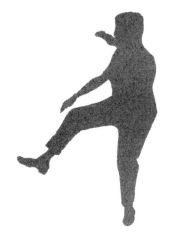

THE THREE CLASSIC WRITINGS ON TAI CHI

❦ The three treatises which follow are considered the basic texts which have come down to us for understanding the essentials of the exercise.

Because they are so lively and helpful and to the point, even the modern student who is learning Tai Chi for his health and well-being, quite without regard to its original background, will want to read them. Delightfully expressed, the treatises often encompass in a few oblique words something that a Westerner would feel obliged to put forth only in extended discussion. The fruit of a whole lifetime's practice is sometimes contained in a single phrase.

As you read along for the first time, skim these pages for whatever pointers and tips on how to do the exercise may have personal meaning for you. Other material that might be of lesser interest to you can on this first reading be skipped entirely.

But return to the three treatises from time to time during your practice of Tai Chi. With increasing experience, you will be able to get more and more from the down-to-earth advice that is being offered there by the great experts who wrote them.

❖   ❖   ❖

I. A Discussion on the Practice of Tai Chi Chuan
(*Traditional. Sometimes attributed to Chang San-feng, 13th Century. See pages 181-184.*)

In each movement the entire body must be light and it is especially important that all parts of the body string together flexibly.

The spirit should withdraw and gather (remain in calm concentration).

Do not allow gaps; do not allow unevenness; do not allow discontinuities.

Your feet are the root, the energy passes through your legs, control is in the waist, and form emerges in your hands and fingers. Advance and retreat in accord with opportunity and conditions of strength.

When opportunity and conditions of strength are not grasped, the body is scattered and in disorder; then the fault must be sought in the waist and in the legs. Up or down, forward or backward, left or right, in all movements this fault is to be guarded against.

All of these comments describe the essential idea, and not merely the externals.

When there is up, there must be down; when there is forward, there must be backward; when there is left, there must be right. If the idea is toward moving upward, hold at the same time the idea of a downward return. For if upon lifting an opposing force you add the idea of pushing it down, then the root of your opposition is broken, and without doubt you will overcome it quickly.

The empty and the solid should be clearly distinguished. Each physical situation by nature has an empty side and a solid side. This is true of every physical situation.

The entire body is strung together, let there not be the slightest break.

❧

II. The Treatise on Tai Chi Chuan
(Attributed to the foremost pupil of Chang San-feng—named Wang Chung-yueh—who lived during the era 1368 A.D. to 1644 A.D. See pages 187 and 190.)

NOTE: For the references in this and the succeeding paper to "the other" and to "combat" it might be well to reread on page 181 the discussion given there of the concept of "chuan," which does not simply mean a physical fight, but may also apply in a wider context.

Tai Chi as the ultimate form arises out of Wu Chi, the formless.

It is the origin of movement and quietude, and the mother of Yin and Yang.

In movement it opens, in quietude it closes.

Without ever exceeding or falling short, Tai Chi moves in bending and stretching.

When I yield to a hard force this is called "moving away."

When I take on a hard force this is called "sticking" with it.

When the other's movement comes quickly, I respond quickly.

When the other's movement comes slowly, I follow slowly,. In a myriad of changing situations, the principle is the same.

From familiarity with the exercise there comes a gradual realization and understanding of force; from the understanding of force there comes a spiritual illumination.

But it is only after long diligent practice that this sudden seeing-through will be achieved.

Empty, alert, still, and quiet.

The breath sinks toward the solar plexus.

Not inclined, not leaning.

Suddenly concealing, suddenly manifesting.

When an intruding weight comes to my left, my left is empty; when an intruding weight comes to my right, then my right disappears.

Looking up, the other feels my height; looking down, the other feels my depth; advancing he feels the distance lengthening; retreating he is more crowded.

A small bird cannot take off; a single fly cannot land.

Others do not know me, but I alone know others.

When great heroes are without match, it is because of all these factors.

There are many other techniques (of combat). Whatever their differences they all nevertheless rely upon the strong to overcome the weak, and the slow to give in to the fast. But as far as the strong beating the weak, the slow giving in to the fast, such things derive from natural abilities and do not have to be studied. When "four ounces move a thousand pounds" it is obviously not a matter of strength. When an old man can withstand many young men, how can it be through an accomplishment of speed?

Stand as a poised scale. In action be as a wheel.

With your center of gravity displaced to one side you can be fluid. If you are "double heavy" [weight evenly distributed on both feet], you become stagnant.

Often one encounters someone who even with many years of study has not achieved proper development and is still subdued by others; this is because he has not realized the fault of "double heaviness."

To avoid this fault, one must know Yin and Yang: to "stick" is also to move away, to move away is also to "stick." Yin does not leave Yang, and Yang does not leave Yin. Yin and Yang always complement each other—to understand this is necessary in order to understand force. (*See the discussion of Yin-Yang influence on Tai Chi, pages 173-174.*)

When one understands force, the more one practices the more wonderful will be his development.
One comprehends in silence and experiences in feeling until gradually one may act at will.

There is the traditional advice, "sacrifice self, follow the other"; but many have misunderstood this to mean abandoning the near in order to seek the far.
A mistake of inches but an error of a thousand leagues! Therefore the student should pay careful heed to what is said.

❦

III.   An Exposition on the Practice of the 13 Movement Forms
(*Attributed to the same authorship as the preceding. See II.*)

NOTE: The 13 movement forms are:
Stepping forward, stepping backward, turning left, turning right, standing centered.
Expanding, drawing, crowding, pressing, gathering, twisting, elbowing, leaning.
In the order listed above these are the five positions and the eight dynamic applications of force which are incorporated in Tai Chi.

The "will"* moves the breath, must order it to sink in, then it can be gathered into the bones.

The breath moves the body, must make it pliable, then it can easily follow the will.

If your energies are picked up, then there is no worry about being sluggish and heavy: to accomplish this your head must feel suspended; but in idea and in breath you must be able to change with alacrity in order to achieve roundness and smoothness of movement; this is accomplished by the interchange of empty and solid.

To deliver force we sink our center of gravity, maintain looseness and quietude, and concentrate in a single direction.

---

* The Chinese word here literally means heart. Some translate it "mind," but mind in Western tradition is devoid of emotions and opposed to the body. Both these implications make it wrong for this word, which will have to be translated at best as "will."

To stand still we remain centrally poised, calm and expanded, and can thus protect ourselves from all eight sides.

To move the breath as fine pearls [an image expressing smallness, roundness and smoothness] there is no place that it does not reach.

To use force as hardened steel, there is no hardness it cannot destroy.

The form is as a hawk catching a rabbit; the spirit, as a cat watching a mouse.

In quietude as the mountain. In movement as the river.

To store force: as if drawing the bow. To issue force: as if releasing the arrow.

Through the curve seek the straight.

First store, then issue.

Strength issues from the back.

Steps follow changes in the body.

To withdraw is to release. To release is to withdraw. To break is to continue.

Back and forth must have folds [no straight path in either case], advancing and retreating must have turns and changes.

Through what is greatly soft one achieves what is greatly hard.

If one is able to inhale and exhale, then one can be light and lively.

Breathing must be nourished without impediment [no holding of the breath and no forcing it], then no harm will come.

Force must be bent [like a bow] and stored, then there is enough to spare.

The "will" orders, the breath goes forth as the banner, the waist takes the command.

First seek to stretch and expand; afterwards seek to tighten and collect; then one attains integrated development.

It is said:
First in the "will," afterwards in the body.

The stomach stays loose. The breath is gathered into the bones. The spirit remains calm.

The body quiet. At every moment remain collected.

It must be remembered; as one part moves, all parts move; if one part is still, all parts are still.

Moving back and forth, the breath goes to the back, gathered toward the spine, making firm the vitality within, but manifesting leisurely calm without.

Step as a cat walks. Use force as if drawing on silk.

Throughout the body the idea rests upon the vitality and not upon the breath; to rest upon the breath causes stagnancy [to guide it, that is, as distinguished from moving the breath, which is to allow it free passage however it may choose to come or go]. To be with breath [holding the breath] is to be without strength. To be without breath [moving the breath, explained above, is likewise called without breath] one can be really strong.

The breath is as the wheel. The waist is as the wheel hub.

It is said:
If the other is not moving, the self does not move.

If the other moves slightly, then the self moves sooner than he.

Seemingly loose, but not loose.

About to stretch but not yet stretched.

The force sometimes stops but the idea continues [what in Western terms is known as the "follow-through"].

❦